ATS-117   ADMISSION TEST SERIES

This is your
PASSBOOK for...

ARRT® Examination in Cardiovascular Interventional Technology (CIT)

Test Preparation Study Guide
Questions & Answers

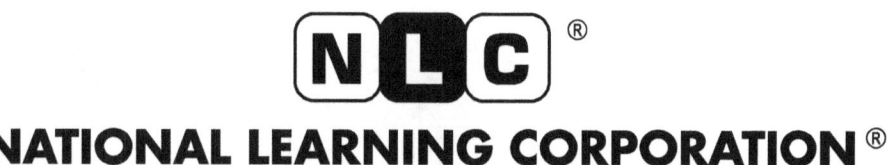

NATIONAL LEARNING CORPORATION®

COPYRIGHT NOTICE

This book is SOLELY intended for, is sold ONLY to, and its use is RESTRICTED to individual, bona fide applicants or candidates who qualify by virtue of having seriously filed applications for appropriate license, certificate, professional and/or promotional advancement, higher school matriculation, scholarship, or other legitimate requirements of education and/or governmental authorities.

This book is NOT intended for use, class instruction, tutoring, training, duplication, copying, reprinting, excerption, or adaptation, etc., by:

1) Other publishers
2) Proprietors and/or Instructors of "Coaching" and/or Preparatory Courses
3) Personnel and/or Training Divisions of commercial, industrial, and governmental organizations
4) Schools, colleges, or universities and/or their departments and staffs, including teachers and other personnel
5) Testing Agencies or Bureaus
6) Study groups which seek by the purchase of a single volume to copy and/or duplicate and/or adapt this material for use by the group as a whole without having purchased individual volumes for each of the members of the group
7) Et al.

Such persons would be in violation of appropriate Federal and State statutes.

PROVISION OF LICENSING AGREEMENTS – Recognized educational, commercial, industrial, and governmental institutions and organizations, and others legitimately engaged in educational pursuits, including training, testing, and measurement activities, may address request for a licensing agreement to the copyright owners, who will determine whether, and under what conditions, including fees and charges, the materials in this book may be used them. In other words, a licensing facility exists for the legitimate use of the material in this book on other than an individual basis. However, it is asseverated and affirmed here that the material in this book CANNOT be used without the receipt of the express permission of such a licensing agreement from the Publishers. Inquiries re licensing should be addressed to the company, attention rights and permissions department.

All rights reserved, including the right of reproduction in whole or in part, in any form or by any means, electronic or mechanical, including photocopying, recording, or by any information storage and retrieval system, without permission in writing from the Publisher.

Copyright © 2024 by
National Learning Corporation

212 Michael Drive, Syosset, NY 11791
(516) 921-8888 • www.passbooks.com
E-mail: info@passbooks.com

PASSBOOK® SERIES

THE *PASSBOOK® SERIES* has been created to prepare applicants and candidates for the ultimate academic battlefield – the examination room.

At some time in our lives, each and every one of us may be required to take an examination – for validation, matriculation, admission, qualification, registration, certification, or licensure.

Based on the assumption that every applicant or candidate has met the basic formal educational standards, has taken the required number of courses, and read the necessary texts, the *PASSBOOK® SERIES* furnishes the one special preparation which may assure passing with confidence, instead of failing with insecurity. Examination questions – together with answers – are furnished as the basic vehicle for study so that the mysteries of the examination and its compounding difficulties may be eliminated or diminished by a sure method.

This book is meant to help you pass your examination provided that you qualify and are serious in your objective.

The entire field is reviewed through the huge store of content information which is succinctly presented through a provocative and challenging approach – the question-and-answer method.

A climate of success is established by furnishing the correct answers at the end of each test.

You soon learn to recognize types of questions, forms of questions, and patterns of questioning. You may even begin to anticipate expected outcomes.

You perceive that many questions are repeated or adapted so that you can gain acute insights, which may enable you to score many sure points.

You learn how to confront new questions, or types of questions, and to attack them confidently and work out the correct answers.

You note objectives and emphases, and recognize pitfalls and dangers, so that you may make positive educational adjustments.

Moreover, you are kept fully informed in relation to new concepts, methods, practices, and directions in the field.

You discover that you are actually taking the examination all the time: you are preparing for the examination by "taking" an examination, not by reading extraneous and/or supererogatory textbooks.

In short, this PASSBOOK®, used directedly, should be an important factor in helping you to pass your test.

ARRT® EXAMINATION IN CARDIOVASCULAR INTERVENTIONAL TECHNOLOGY

INTRODUCTION

The purpose of the ARRT Examination in Cardiovascular Interventional Technology is to assess the knowledge and cognitive skills underlying the intelligent performance of the major tasks typically required of a technologist employed in this specialized area. The Registry performed a job analysis project for the discipline for the purpose of developing the linkage between typical tasks and the examination content. The task inventories and content specifications resulting from that project were utilized for the development of examinations.

While it is recognized that some employment settings focus on only a subpart of the overall domain of tasks, it is desirable that the scope of practice for the cardiovascular-interventional technologist be defined on a broader scale.

Although procedural details may be system-specific, the underlying commonality provided by the general principles of cardiovascular-interventional technology, radiographic imaging, patient care, and the overriding concern for radiation safety, tie cardiovascular-interventional procedures together into a unitary discipline.

It is therefore the opinion of the Registry that a cardiovascular-interventional technologist should be qualified to participate in routine cardiovascular-interventional procedures for all physiological systems as identified in the ARRT Job Analysis Project. It is acknowledged that an orientation period will be necessary for any technologist entering a new setting to become familiar with equipment, protocols and specific procedures which may be somewhat different than those with which the technologist has familiarity.

Test performance will be evaluated as a whole and the creation of categories of recognition for subspecialties within the cardiovascular-interventional technology domain will be avoided.

THE EXAMINATION

The first section of the document outlines the knowledge areas underlying task performance. Category weights are provided for each of the major content categories. The weightings listed for subcategories within the major categories are intended to provide general guidelines for test construction and are subject to some variation across test forms.

HOW TO TAKE A TEST

You have studied long, hard and conscientiously.

With your official admission card in hand, and your heart pounding, you have been admitted to the examination room.

You note that there are several hundred other applicants in the examination room waiting to take the same test.

They all appear to be equally well prepared.

You know that nothing but your best effort will suffice. The "moment of truth" is at hand: you now have to demonstrate objectively, in writing, your knowledge of content and your understanding of subject matter.

You are fighting the most important battle of your life—to pass and/or score high on an examination which will determine your career and provide the economic basis for your livelihood.

What extra, special things should you know and should you do in taking the examination?

I. YOU MUST PASS AN EXAMINATION

A. WHAT EVERY CANDIDATE SHOULD KNOW
Examination applicants often ask us for help in preparing for the written test. What can I study in advance? What kinds of questions will be asked? How will the test be given? How will the papers be graded?

B. HOW ARE EXAMS DEVELOPED?
Examinations are carefully written by trained technicians who are specialists in the field known as "psychological measurement," in consultation with recognized authorities in the field of work that the test will cover. These experts recommend the subject matter areas or skills to be tested; only those knowledges or skills important to your success on the job are included. The most reliable books and source materials available are used as references. Together, the experts and technicians judge the difficulty level of the questions.
Test technicians know how to phrase questions so that the problem is clearly stated. Their ethics do not permit "trick" or "catch" questions. Questions may have been tried out on sample groups, or subjected to statistical analysis, to determine their usefulness.
Written tests are often used in combination with performance tests, ratings of training and experience, and oral interviews. All of these measures combine to form the best-known means of finding the right person for the right job.

II. HOW TO PASS THE WRITTEN TEST

A. BASIC STEPS

1) Study the announcement

How, then, can you know what subjects to study? Our best answer is: "Learn as much as possible about the class of positions for which you've applied." The exam will test the knowledge, skills and abilities needed to do the work.

Your most valuable source of information about the position you want is the official exam announcement. This announcement lists the training and experience qualifications. Check these standards and apply only if you come reasonably close to meeting them. Many jurisdictions preview the written test in the exam announcement by including a section called "Knowledge and Abilities Required," "Scope of the Examination," or some similar heading. Here you will find out specifically what fields will be tested.

2) Choose appropriate study materials

If the position for which you are applying is technical or advanced, you will read more advanced, specialized material. If you are already familiar with the basic principles of your field, elementary textbooks would waste your time. Concentrate on advanced textbooks and technical periodicals. Think through the concepts and review difficult problems in your field.

These are all general sources. You can get more ideas on your own initiative, following these leads. For example, training manuals and publications of the government agency which employs workers in your field can be useful, particularly for technical and professional positions. A letter or visit to the government department involved may result in more specific study suggestions, and certainly will provide you with a more definite idea of the exact nature of the position you are seeking.

3) Study this book!

III. KINDS OF TESTS

Tests are used for purposes other than measuring knowledge and ability to perform specified duties. For some positions, it is equally important to test ability to make adjustments to new situations or to profit from training. In others, basic mental abilities not dependent on information are essential. Questions which test these things may not appear as pertinent to the duties of the position as those which test for knowledge and information. Yet they are often highly important parts of a fair examination. For very general questions, it is almost impossible to help you direct your study efforts. What we can do is to point out some of the more common of these general abilities needed in public service positions and describe some typical questions.

1) General information

Broad, general information has been found useful for predicting job success in some kinds of work. This is tested in a variety of ways, from vocabulary lists to questions about current events. Basic background in some field of work, such as sociology or economics, may be sampled in a group of questions. Often these are principles which have become familiar to most persons through exposure rather than through formal training. It is difficult to advise you how to study for these questions; being alert to the world around you is our best suggestion.

2) Verbal ability

An example of an ability needed in many positions is verbal or language ability. Verbal ability is, in brief, the ability to use and understand words. Vocabulary and grammar tests are typical measures of this ability. Reading comprehension or paragraph interpretation questions are common in many kinds of civil service tests. You are given a paragraph of written material and asked to find its central meaning.

IV. KINDS OF QUESTIONS

1. Multiple-choice Questions

Most popular of the short-answer questions is the "multiple choice" or "best answer" question. It can be used, for example, to test for factual knowledge, ability to solve problems or judgment in meeting situations found at work.

A multiple-choice question is normally one of three types:
- It can begin with an incomplete statement followed by several possible endings. You are to find the one ending which best completes the statement, although some of the others may not be entirely wrong.
- It can also be a complete statement in the form of a question which is answered by choosing one of the statements listed.
- It can be in the form of a problem – again you select the best answer.

Here is an example of a multiple-choice question with a discussion which should give you some clues as to the method for choosing the right answer:

When an employee has a complaint about his assignment, the action which will best help him overcome his difficulty is to
- A. discuss his difficulty with his coworkers
- B. take the problem to the head of the organization
- C. take the problem to the person who gave him the assignment
- D. say nothing to anyone about his complaint

In answering this question, you should study each of the choices to find which is best. Consider choice "A" – Certainly an employee may discuss his complaint with fellow employees, but no change or improvement can result, and the complaint remains unresolved. Choice "B" is a poor choice since the head of the organization probably does not know what assignment you have been given, and taking your problem to him is known as "going over the head" of the supervisor. The supervisor, or person who made the assignment, is the person who can clarify it or correct any injustice. Choice "C" is, therefore, correct. To say nothing, as in choice "D," is unwise. Supervisors have and interest in knowing the problems employees are facing, and the employee is seeking a solution to his problem.

2. True/False

3. Matching Questions

Matching an answer from a column of choices within another column.

V. RECORDING YOUR ANSWERS

Computer terminals are used more and more today for many different kinds of exams.

For an examination with very few applicants, you may be told to record your answers in the test booklet itself. Separate answer sheets are much more common. If this separate answer sheet is to be scored by machine – and this is often the case – it is highly important that you mark your answers correctly in order to get credit.

VI. BEFORE THE TEST

YOUR PHYSICAL CONDITION IS IMPORTANT

If you are not well, you can't do your best work on tests. If you are half asleep, you can't do your best either. Here are some tips:

1) Get about the same amount of sleep you usually get. Don't stay up all night before the test, either partying or worrying—DON'T DO IT!
2) If you wear glasses, be sure to wear them when you go to take the test. This goes for hearing aids, too.
3) If you have any physical problems that may keep you from doing your best, be sure to tell the person giving the test. If you are sick or in poor health, you relay cannot do your best on any test. You can always come back and take the test some other time.

Common sense will help you find procedures to follow to get ready for an examination. Too many of us, however, overlook these sensible measures. Indeed, nervousness and fatigue have been found to be the most serious reasons why applicants fail to do their best on civil service tests. Here is a list of reminders:

- Begin your preparation early – Don't wait until the last minute to go scurrying around for books and materials or to find out what the position is all about.
- Prepare continuously – An hour a night for a week is better than an all-night cram session. This has been definitely established. What is more, a night a week for a month will return better dividends than crowding your study into a shorter period of time.
- Locate the place of the exam – You have been sent a notice telling you when and where to report for the examination. If the location is in a different town or otherwise unfamiliar to you, it would be well to inquire the best route and learn something about the building.
- Relax the night before the test – Allow your mind to rest. Do not study at all that night. Plan some mild recreation or diversion; then go to bed early and get a good night's sleep.
- Get up early enough to make a leisurely trip to the place for the test – This way unforeseen events, traffic snarls, unfamiliar buildings, etc. will not upset you.
- Dress comfortably – A written test is not a fashion show. You will be known by number and not by name, so wear something comfortable.
- Leave excess paraphernalia at home – Shopping bags and odd bundles will get in your way. You need bring only the items mentioned in the official notice you received; usually everything you need is provided. Do not bring reference books to the exam. They will only confuse those last minutes and be taken away from you when in the test room.

- Arrive somewhat ahead of time – If because of transportation schedules you must get there very early, bring a newspaper or magazine to take your mind off yourself while waiting.
- Locate the examination room – When you have found the proper room, you will be directed to the seat or part of the room where you will sit. Sometimes you are given a sheet of instructions to read while you are waiting. Do not fill out any forms until you are told to do so; just read them and be prepared.
- Relax and prepare to listen to the instructions
- If you have any physical problem that may keep you from doing your best, be sure to tell the test administrator. If you are sick or in poor health, you really cannot do your best on the exam. You can come back and take the test some other time.

VII. AT THE TEST

The day of the test is here and you have the test booklet in your hand. The temptation to get going is very strong. Caution! There is more to success than knowing the right answers. You must know how to identify your papers and understand variations in the type of short-answer question used in this particular examination. Follow these suggestions for maximum results from your efforts:

1) Cooperate with the monitor

The test administrator has a duty to create a situation in which you can be as much at ease as possible. He will give instructions, tell you when to begin, check to see that you are marking your answer sheet correctly, and so on. He is not there to guard you, although he will see that your competitors do not take unfair advantage. He wants to help you do your best.

2) Listen to all instructions

Don't jump the gun! Wait until you understand all directions. In most civil service tests you get more time than you need to answer the questions. So don't be in a hurry. Read each word of instructions until you clearly understand the meaning. Study the examples, listen to all announcements and follow directions. Ask questions if you do not understand what to do.

3) Identify your papers

Civil service exams are usually identified by number only. You will be assigned a number; you must not put your name on your test papers. Be sure to copy your number correctly. Since more than one exam may be given, copy your exact examination title.

4) Plan your time

Unless you are told that a test is a "speed" or "rate of work" test, speed itself is usually not important. Time enough to answer all the questions will be provided, but this does not mean that you have all day. An overall time limit has been set. Divide the total time (in minutes) by the number of questions to determine the approximate time you have for each question.

5) Do not linger over difficult questions

If you come across a difficult question, mark it with a paper clip (useful to have along) and come back to it when you have been through the booklet. One caution if you do this – be sure to skip a number on your answer sheet as well. Check often to be sure that you have not lost your place and that you are marking in the row numbered the same as the question you are answering.

6) Read the questions

Be sure you know what the question asks! Many capable people are unsuccessful because they failed to read the questions correctly.

7) Answer all questions

Unless you have been instructed that a penalty will be deducted for incorrect answers, it is better to guess than to omit a question.

8) Speed tests

It is often better NOT to guess on speed tests. It has been found that on timed tests people are tempted to spend the last few seconds before time is called in marking answers at random – without even reading them – in the hope of picking up a few extra points. To discourage this practice, the instructions may warn you that your score will be "corrected" for guessing. That is, a penalty will be applied. The incorrect answers will be deducted from the correct ones, or some other penalty formula will be used.

9) Review your answers

If you finish before time is called, go back to the questions you guessed or omitted to give them further thought. Review other answers if you have time.

10) Return your test materials

If you are ready to leave before others have finished or time is called, take ALL your materials to the monitor and leave quietly. Never take any test material with you. The monitor can discover whose papers are not complete, and taking a test booklet may be grounds for disqualification.

VIII. EXAMINATION TECHNIQUES

1) Read the general instructions carefully. These are usually printed on the first page of the exam booklet. As a rule, these instructions refer to the timing of the examination; the fact that you should not start work until the signal and must stop work at a signal, etc. If there are any special instructions, such as a choice of questions to be answered, make sure that you note this instruction carefully.

2) When you are ready to start work on the examination, that is as soon as the signal has been given, read the instructions to each question booklet, underline any key words or phrases, such as least, best, outline, describe and the like. In this way you will tend to answer as requested rather than discover on reviewing your paper that you listed without describing, that you selected the worst choice rather than the best choice, etc.

3) If the examination is of the objective or multiple-choice type – that is, each question will also give a series of possible answers: A, B, C or D, and you are called upon to select the best answer and write the letter next to that answer on your answer paper – it is advisable to start answering each question in turn. There may be anywhere from 50 to 100 such questions in the three or four hours allotted and you can see how much time would be taken if you read through all the questions before beginning to answer any. Furthermore, if you

come across a question or group of questions which you know would be difficult to answer, it would undoubtedly affect your handling of all the other questions.

4) If the examination is of the essay type and contains but a few questions, it is a moot point as to whether you should read all the questions before starting to answer any one. Of course, if you are given a choice – say five out of seven and the like – then it is essential to read all the questions so you can eliminate the two that are most difficult. If, however, you are asked to answer all the questions, there may be danger in trying to answer the easiest one first because you may find that you will spend too much time on it. The best technique is to answer the first question, then proceed to the second, etc.

5) Time your answers. Before the exam begins, write down the time it started, then add the time allowed for the examination and write down the time it must be completed, then divide the time available somewhat as follows:
    - If 3-1/2 hours are allowed, that would be 210 minutes. If you have 80 objective-type questions, that would be an average of 2-1/2 minutes per question. Allow yourself no more than 2 minutes per question, or a total of 160 minutes, which will permit about 50 minutes to review.
    - If for the time allotment of 210 minutes there are 7 essay questions to answer, that would average about 30 minutes a question. Give yourself only 25 minutes per question so that you have about 35 minutes to review.

6) The most important instruction is to read each question and make sure you know what is wanted. The second most important instruction is to time yourself properly so that you answer every question. The third most important instruction is to answer every question. Guess if you have to but include something for each question. Remember that you will receive no credit for a blank and will probably receive some credit if you write something in answer to an essay question. If you guess a letter – say "B" for a multiple-choice question – you may have guessed right. If you leave a blank as an answer to a multiple-choice question, the examiners may respect your feelings but it will not add a point to your score. Some exams may penalize you for wrong answers, so in such cases only, you may not want to guess unless you have some basis for your answer.

7) Suggestions
    a. Objective-type questions
        1. Examine the question booklet for proper sequence of pages and questions
        2. Read all instructions carefully
        3. Skip any question which seems too difficult; return to it after all other questions have been answered
        4. Apportion your time properly; do not spend too much time on any single question or group of questions
        5. Note and underline key words – all, most, fewest, least, best, worst, same, opposite, etc.
        6. Pay particular attention to negatives
        7. Note unusual option, e.g., unduly long, short, complex, different or similar in content to the body of the question
        8. Observe the use of "hedging" words – probably, may, most likely, etc.

9. Make sure that your answer is put next to the same number as the question
10. Do not second-guess unless you have good reason to believe the second answer is definitely more correct
11. Cross out original answer if you decide another answer is more accurate; do not erase until you are ready to hand your paper in
12. Answer all questions; guess unless instructed otherwise
13. Leave time for review

b. Essay questions
1. Read each question carefully
2. Determine exactly what is wanted. Underline key words or phrases.
3. Decide on outline or paragraph answer
4. Include many different points and elements unless asked to develop any one or two points or elements
5. Show impartiality by giving pros and cons unless directed to select one side only
6. Make and write down any assumptions you find necessary to answer the questions
7. Watch your English, grammar, punctuation and choice of words
8. Time your answers; don't crowd material

8) Answering the essay question

Most essay questions can be answered by framing the specific response around several key words or ideas. Here are a few such key words or ideas:

M's: manpower, materials, methods, money, management
P's: purpose, program, policy, plan, procedure, practice, problems, pitfalls, personnel, public relations

a. Six basic steps in handling problems:
1. Preliminary plan and background development
2. Collect information, data and facts
3. Analyze and interpret information, data and facts
4. Analyze and develop solutions as well as make recommendations
5. Prepare report and sell recommendations
6. Install recommendations and follow up effectiveness

b. Pitfalls to avoid
1. Taking things for granted – A statement of the situation does not necessarily imply that each of the elements is necessarily true; for example, a complaint may be invalid and biased so that all that can be taken for granted is that a complaint has been registered
2. Considering only one side of a situation – Wherever possible, indicate several alternatives and then point out the reasons you selected the best one
3. Failing to indicate follow up – Whenever your answer indicates action on your part, make certain that you will take proper follow-up action to see how successful your recommendations, procedures or actions turn out to be
4. Taking too long in answering any single question – Remember to time your answers properly

EXAMINATION SECTION

CHARACTERIZATION SECTION

EXAMINATION SECTION
TEST 1

DIRECTIONS: Each question or incomplete statement is followed by several suggested answers or completions. Select the one that BEST answers the question or completes the statement. *PRINT THE LETTER OF THE CORRECT ANSWER IN THE SPACE AT THE RIGHT.*

1. Which of the following decrease in size as they get farther away from the heart? 1.____
   A. Arteries   B. Veins   C. Capillaries   D. Venules

2. Which of the following return deoxygenated blood from the body to the right side of the heart and increase in size as they get closer to the heart? 2.____
   A. Arteries   B. Veins   C. Capillaries   D. Venules

3. All of the following are characteristics of the left main artery EXCEPT: 3.____
   A. Supplies anterior circulation
   B. Arises from the root of the aorta
   C. Short segment
   D. Supplies at least 70% of blood to the myocardium

4. The Sinus of _____ is considered to be the root of the aorta. 4.____
   A. Oddi   B. Morgagni   C. Valsalva   D. Mehta

5. All of the following are characteristics of the left anterior descending artery EXCEPT: 5.____
   A. First branch of the left main
   B. Supplies anterior circulation
   C. Travels toward the base of the heart
   D. Branches into diagonals

6. The circumflex artery is a branch of the _____ artery. 6.____
   A. posterior descending   B. left anterior descending
   C. right coronary   D. left main

7. All of the following are characteristics of the circumflex artery EXCEPT: 7.____
   A. Second branch of the left main coronary artery
   B. Travels posteriorly to the back of the heart
   C. Joins the left coronary through anastomosis
   D. Has one branch

8. The _____ artery is a branch of the circumflex artery. 8.____
   A. left marginal   B. left anterior descending
   C. right marginal   D. posterior descending

9. The _____ artery branches into the posterior descending artery.
   A. left main coronary
   B. left anterior descending
   C. right coronary
   B. circumflex

10. The _____ is located at the root of the aorta and is the origin of the right and left coronary arteries.
    A. aortic arch
    B. ascending aorta
    C. bulb
    D. superior vena cava

11. Which of the following travels superiorly from the bulb and arches posteriorly?
    A. Aortic arch
    B. Ascending aorta
    C. Superior vena cava
    D. Inferior vena cava

12. All of the following are branches of the aortic arch EXCEPT
    A. brachiocephalic artery
    B. left common carotid artery
    C. left subclavian artery
    D. right common carotid artery

13. All of the following are variations of the aortic arch EXCEPT
    A. left circumflex aorta
    B. inverse aorta
    C. prolapsed aorta
    D. pseudocoarctation

14. What blood vessel is the continuation of the thoracic aorta, lies anterior of the vertebral column, and extends from the level of the diaphragm to the L4 vertebra?
    A. Abdominal aorta
    B. Celiac axis
    C. Superior mesenteric artery
    D. Inferior mesenteric artery

15. All of the following are branches of the abdominal aorta EXCEPT
    A. celiac axis
    B. right renal artery
    C. left renal artery
    D. splenic artery

16. The celiac axis originates at what vertebral level?
    A. T4   B. T8   C. T12   D. L2

17. All of the following are branches of the celiac axis EXCEPT
    A. hepatic artery
    B. splenic artery
    C. left gastric artery
    D. left renal artery

18. The superior mesenteric artery originates at what vertebral level?
    A. T8   B. T10   C. L1   D. L5

19. The superior mesenteric artery supplies blood to all of the following EXCEPT
    A. cecum
    B. ascending colon
    C. descending colon
    D. small bowel

20. The inferior mesenteric artery originates at what vertebral level?
    A. T12   B. L3   C. L5   D. S3

21. The inferior mesenteric artery supplies blood to all of the following EXCEPT   21.____
    A. sigmoid colon   B. hepatic flexure
    C. splenic flexure   D. descending colon

22. The left _____ artery arises directly from the aortic arch, the right originates   22.____
    from the brachiocephalic artery, and both pass laterally under the clavicle.
    A. subclavian   B. vertebral   C. axillary   D. brachial

23. The subclavian artery turns into the _____ artery at the lateral border of the   23.____
    first rib.
    A. axillary   B. brachial   C. radial   D. ulnar

24. The _____, also called the brachiocephalic artery, is the first branch from   24.____
    the aortic arch after the ascending aorta, travels superiorly to the right, and is a
    very short segment.
    A. invertebral artery   B. innominate artery
    C. left common carotid   D. left subclavian

25. The innominate artery is responsible for all of the following types of   25.____
    circulation EXCEPT _____ circulation.
    A. anterior cerebral   B. posterior cerebral
    C. upper extremity   D. systemic

KEY (CORRECT ANSWERS)

1.	A		11.	B
2.	B		12.	D
3.	A		13.	C
4.	C		14.	A
5.	C		15.	D
6.	D		16.	C
7.	C		17.	D
8.	A		18.	C
9.	C		19.	C
10.	C		20.	B

21.	B
22.	A
23.	A
24.	B
25.	D

TEST 2

DIRECTIONS: Each question or incomplete statement is followed by several suggested answers or completions. Select the one that BEST answers the question or completes the statement. *PRINT THE LETTER OF THE CORRECT ANSWER IN THE SPACE AT THE RIGHT.*

1. The external carotids are responsible for blood supply to all of the following EXCEPT
   A. pituitary gland
   B. scalp
   C. face
   D. anterior neck

   1.____

2. The internal carotids are responsible for blood supply to all of the following EXCEPT
   A. anterior intercranial tissue
   B. pituitary gland
   C. orbits
   D. meninges

   2.____

3. The internal carotids form an "S" shape that is commonly known as the carotid
   A. structures   B. siphon   C. pathway   D. tunnel

   3.____

4. Hypaque contrast material is _____ and causes an immediate decrease in cardiac output following administration.
   A. isotonic   B. hypertonic   C. hypotonic   D. epitonic

   4.____

5. Which of the following is the chemical element in contrast material that precipitates it being radiopaque when exposed to x-rays?
   A. Bromine   B. Iodine   C. Alanine   D. Guanine

   5.____

6. What quality among newer contrast agents such as Hexabrix and Omnipaque allow them not to overload blood volume for a patient in congestive heart failure?
   A. Increased ionization
   B. Low osmolarity
   C. Low iodine content
   D. Low sodium content

   6.____

7. Abnormal left ventricular function is commonly considered to be a cardiac ejection fraction less than
   A. 30%   B. 40%   C. 50%   D. 70%

   7.____

8. What is the common term for left ventricular walls that act like aneurysms and bulge during systole?
   A. Akinetic
   B. Dyskinetic
   C. Hyperkinetic
   D. Hypokinetic

   8.____

9. Which of the following should be used to inflate the balloon when performing a right heart catheterization on a cyanotic child?
   A. Contrast/Saline mixture
   B. Sterile saline
   C. Nitrous oxide
   D. Carbon dioxide

   9.____

10. A Swan-Ganz balloon should NEVER be filled with
    A. oxygen
    B. carbon dioxide
    C. contrast
    D. sterile saline

11. When performing an invasive procedure, the balloon should be inflated in the
    A. femoral vein
    B. inferior vena cava
    C. right ventricle
    D. left atrium

12. The tip in the _____ is the MOST stable place to leave a right heart catheter positioned.
    A. pulmonary artery wedge
    B. pulmonary artery
    C. right ventricle
    D. right atrium

13. When wedging a Swan-Ganz catheter, which of the following would be APPROPRIATE in order to prevent rupture of the pulmonary artery?
    A. Always use 1.5ml of air to inflate the balloon for a pulmonary occlusion pressure.
    B. Advance PAC slightly if pulmonary artery occlusion pressure waveform is obtained with less than 1.25ml of air.
    C. Withdraw PAC slightly if pulmonary artery occlusion pressure waveform is obtained with less than 1.25ml of air.
    D. Frequently monitor pulmonary artery occlusion pressure.

14. Which of the following statements is TRUE regarding clot formation on Swan-Ganz catheters?
    A. Heparin should be added to IV solutions for all patients with a Swan-Ganz catheter.
    B. Catheters with clot formation should be flushed extensively with saline.
    C. Clot formation begins after 3-5 days in the vessel.
    D. All intravascular monitoring catheters are at risk for clot formation.

15. What action should be performed prior to withdrawing a Swan-Ganz catheter to record PA-RV pressures?
    A. Deflate the balloon.
    B. Inflate the balloon.
    C. Distal lumen should be flushed.
    D. Proximal lumen should be flushed.

16. Which of the following statements is TRUE regarding abnormal central venous O_2 saturation?
    A. SvO2 values <0.60 indicate threatened tissue oxygenation.
    B. SvO2 values >0.80 indicate adequate tissue oxygenation.
    C. SvO2 values <0.60 indicate low oxygen consumption.
    D. SvO2 values >0.80 indicate increased oxygen consumption.

17. Central venous pressure can directly assess which of the following?
    A. RV function and LV function
    B. RV function and fluid volume status
    C. LV function and myocardial contractility
    D. Fluid volume status and myocardial contractility

18. Hypovolemia is MOST commonly associated with
    A. decreased heart rate
    B. increased central venous pressure
    C. decreased RV end-diastolic pressure
    D. increased PA occlusion pressure

19. Which of the following statements is TRUE regarding pulmonary artery occlusion wedge pressure?
    A. Is measured through the most proximal catheter port
    B. The waveform always contains three positive waves
    C. Changes to a right ventricular waveform during the inflation of the balloon
    D. Blood flow is stopped creating a static column of blood between the tip and the left atrium

20. Which of the following statements is TRUE regarding hemodynamic waveforms?
    A. Rises during inspiration for a patient breathing spontaneously
    B. Falls during inspiration for a patient on a ventilator
    C. Should be read at point of end expiration for a patient breathing spontaneously
    D. Should be read at peak-inspiration for a patient on a ventilator

21. For what reason are large holes cut into the sides of PTCA guider catheters?
    A. Even disbursement of contrast media
    B. Reduce trauma and dissection of coronary ostium
    C. Prevent catheter damping
    D. To allow initiation of a second guide wire

22. What substance is used in the construction of the majority of balloon floatation catheters because it has the least memory and torque control?
    A. Teflon   B. Polyurethane
    C. Polyethylene   D. Poly vinyl chloride

23. In the United States, what type of cardiac catheters are permitted to be resterilized by third party reprocessor companies?
    A. PTCA balloon catheters   B. Polyurethane catheters
    C. Teflon catheters   D. Electrophysiology electrodes

24. Which of the following is the major DISADVANTAGE of using angiographic flood catheters with multiple side holes?   24.____
    A. Trauma to blood vessel walls
    B. Increased frequency of clot formation
    C. Cannot be used with leading guidewire
    D. Trauma to intracardiac valves

25. Optimal WEDGE pressures can be obtained only through the use of which of the following catheters?   25.____
    A. End-hole only
    B. Four side holes
    C. Four side holes + end hole
    D. Six side holes + distal balloon

KEY (CORRECT ANSWERS)

1.	A		11.	B
2.	D		12.	B
3.	B		13.	C
4.	B		14.	D
5.	B		15.	A
6.	B		16.	A
7.	C		17.	B
8.	B		18.	C
9.	D		19.	D
10.	C		20.	C

21.	C
22.	D
23.	D
24.	B
25.	A

TEST 3

DIRECTIONS: Each question or incomplete statement is followed by several suggested answers or completions. Select the one that BEST answers the question or completes the statement. *PRINT THE LETTER OF THE CORRECT ANSWER IN THE SPACE AT THE RIGHT.*

1. What type of catheter is designed for hemodynamic measurements only and not designed for angiography due to excessive kickback with rapid injection?
    A. Multipurpose/Gensini
    B. Pigtail/Van Tassel Pigtail
    C. Lehmand/Cornand
    D. NIH/Berman

    1.____

2. Due to increased stability and no end hole, which of the following is the PREFERRED right heart angiographic catheter for infants and children?
    A. Multipurpose/Gensini
    B. Pigtail/Van Tassel Pigtail
    C. Lehmand/Cornand
    D. NIH/Berman

    2.____

3. Multipurpose catheters should NOT be injected into at rates exceeding
    A. 2ml/sec   B. 5ml/sec   C. 8ml/sec   D. 10ml/sec

    3.____

4. What is the recommended bodily position for a patient suffering from pulmonary edema?
    A. Prone   B. Supine   C. Upright   D. Trendelenburg

    4.____

5. Catheters with a closed end may be introduced through all of the following methods EXCEPT
    A. Seldinger over-the-wire
    B. femoral cutdown
    C. brachial cutdown
    D. femoral sheath

    5.____

6. In advance of performing any cardiac invasive procedure, who carries the responsibility of obtaining informed consent?
    A. Nurse assisting with the procedure
    B. Technologist assisting with the procedure
    C. Primary care physician
    D. Physician performing the procedure

    6.____

7. What is the purpose of obtaining informed consent?
    A. To authorize all routine hospital procedures
    B. Protect patient from unnecessary high risk procedures
    C. Protect performing physician and hospital from claims of an unauthorized medical procedure
    C. Authorize physician to withhold lifesaving treatment if appropriate

    7.____

8. All of the following are risk factors for acute myocardial infarction EXCEPT
    A. high estrogen levels
    B. diabetes
    C. hypertension
    D. elevated lipids

    8.____

9. What childhood illness will predispose an individual to develop a heart murmur?
   A. Measles
   B. Mumps
   C. Rheumatic fever
   D. Chickenpox

10. According to Universal or Standard precautions, in emergency situations, what body fluids are considered to be infectious?
    A. All body fluids of all patients
    B. All body fluids of infected patients
    C. Blood and certain body fluids of all patients
    D. Blood and certain body fluids of infected patients

11. What should be the FIRST medication administered to all ACLS patients?
    A. Aspirin   B. Oxygen   C. Heparin   D. Nitroglycerin

12. All of the following are advantages to using vasopressin over epinephrine treatment of ventricular fibrillation and pulseless ventricular tachycardia EXCEPT
    A. reduced cardiac ischemia and irritability
    B. shorter half-life
    C. one time dose
    D. reduced risk of ventricular fibrillation

13. What vitamin is required for the formation of clotting factors?
    A. A   B. B12   C. D   D. K

14. A patient was given 5,000 units of heparin prior to a cardiac catheterization. The performing physician wishes to neutralize 4,000 units of heparin. What would be the APPROPRIATE intervention to neutralize 4,000 units of heparin?
    A. 200mcg Protamine
    B. 40mg Protamine
    C. 20mcg Amicar
    D. 40mg Amicar

15. Which of the following is a cardiac-specific serum biomarker released from damaged myocardial tissue cells?
    A. Troponin T   B. Troponin I   C. Myoglobin   D. CK

16. Which biomarker is non-specific, used in conjunction with others, appears in both cardiac and skeletal muscle, and begins rising 1-4 hours post myocardial infarction?
    A. Troponin T   B. Troponin I   C. Myoglobin   D. CK

17. How long does it take Troponin I serum biomarker to return to baseline?
    A. 3-12 hours
    B. 12-48 hours
    C. 48-96 hours
    D. 5-10 days

18. What are the two basic tests that would be performed if a patient was complaining of chest pain?
    A. Chest x-ray and EKG
    B. EKG and echocardiogram
    C. Stress test and echocardiogram
    D. EKG and cardiac catheterization

19. All of the following are methods of hemodynamic monitoring performed at the bedside EXCEPT
    A. arterial catheter
    B. central venous pressure catheter
    C. PICC line
    D. Pulmonary artery catheterization

20. Normal cardiac output is _____ L/min.
    A. 1-2   B. 2-4   C. 3-6   D. 4-8

21. The amount of blood the right ventricle and left ventricle pump per contraction is referred to as
    A. cardiac output
    B. stroke volume
    C. blood pressure
    D. blood volume

22. Normal stroke volume is _____ mL/beat.
    A. 25-50   B. 40-80   C. 60-130   D. 80-150

23. Which of the following is defined as an increase in preload, myocardial stretch, and force of contraction will increase stroke volume?
    A. Ohm's Law
    B. Frank-Starling Law
    C. Starks Law
    D. Law of Laplace

24. All of the following are able to increase the contractility of the heart EXCEPT
    A. potassium   B. calcium   C. caffeine   D. digitalis

25. _____ is defined as the degree of vascular resistance impeding the ventricular ejection of blood.
    A. Preload
    B. Afterload
    C. Stroke volume
    D. Contractility

KEY (CORRECT ANSWERS)

1. C
2. D
3. D
4. C
5. A

6. D
7. C
8. A
9. C
10. A

11. B
12. B
13. D
14. B
15. B

16. C
17. D
18. A
19. C
20. D

21. B
22. C
23. B
24. A
25. B

TEST 4

DIRECTIONS: Each question or incomplete statement is followed by several suggested answers or completions. Select the one that BEST answers the question or completes the statement. *PRINT THE LETTER OF THE CORRECT ANSWER IN THE SPACE AT THE RIGHT.*

1. What is the MOST common side effect associated with cardiac catheterization? 1._____
   A. Hypotension
   B. Anaphylaxis
   C. Bleeding at the puncture site
   D. Myocardial infarction

2. What aspect of the QRS complex represents vascular repolarization? 2._____
   A. P-wave
   B. PR-interval
   C. QT-interval
   D. T-wave

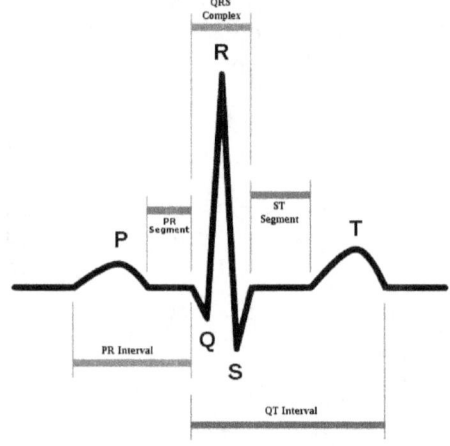

3. Which of the following blood pressures would contraindicate angiography? 3._____
   A. 90/60 mmHg
   B. 110/80 mmHg
   C. 120/90 mmHg
   D. 150/100 mmHg

4. Which of the following is used to measure ventricular pressures? 4._____
   A. EKG
   B. Transducer
   C. Oximeter
   D. Manifold

5. Which medication could be used to relax the arterial walls during angiography? 5._____
   A. Benadryl
   B. Nitroglycerin
   C. Demerol
   D. Pitressin

6. Which medication would be beneficial in an emergency situation in which the patient is experiencing multiple PVC's? 6._____
   A. Lidocaine
   B. Verapamil
   C. Calcium chloride
   D. Sodium chloride

7. Which of the following pulse points requires the use of a stethoscope? 7._____
   A. Popliteal
   B. Brachial
   C. Apical
   D. Femoral

8. Which medical condition arises from acute compression of the heart from fluid that prevents the heart from expanding causing an increased heart rate and decreased blood pressure? 8._____
   A. Pericarditis
   B. Endocarditis
   C. Cardiac tamponade
   D. Congestive heart failure

9. An aortagram or a venacavogram would MOST likely require the use of a _____ catheter.
   A. Pigtail   B. Grollman   C. Sones   D. Amplatz

10. For a cine image to appear dynamic, the minimum frame rate is _____ frames/sec.
    A. 4   B. 8   C. 12   D. 16

11. All of the following catheters are appropriate for coronary angiography EXCEPT
    A. Van Aman   B. Judkins   C. Amplatz   D. Sones

12. What method of digital subtraction angiography enhancement is used to compensate for patient motion?
    A. Pixel shifting
    B. Edge enhancement
    C. Image zoom
    D. Landmarking

13. The gate of a cine camera refers to the
    A. aperture
    B. exposure area
    C. rotating shutter
    D. takeup spool

14. Which medication is required for drug eluting stents?
    A. Heparin   B. Plavix   C. Digoxin   D. Metoprolol

15. What technique is MOST commonly used for performing invasive angiography?
    A. Debakey   B. Evans   C. Seldinger   D. Schrodinger

16. The national safety goal of getting myocardial infarction patients to a cardiac catheterization laboratory is within _____ minutes.
    A. 15   B. 30   C. 60   D. 90

17. Which medications should NOT be taken prior to a cardiac catheterization procedure?
    A. Metoprolol and Verapamil
    B. Digoxin and Nitroglycerin
    C. Imdur and Lisinopril
    D. Metformin and Coumadin

18. Intracoronary radiation via seeds or liquid filled balloons is referred to as
    A. brachytherapy
    B. laser angioplasty
    C. arthrectomy
    D. cardioversion

19. Which of the following is a short-term venous access inserted by direct percutaneous puncture and advanced under fluoroscopic guidance?
    A. Arterial catheter
    B. Central venous pressure catheter
    C. PICC line
    D. Pulmonary artery catheterization

20. Which projection would be used to properly visualize the aortic arch?   20._____
    A. AP   B. Lateral   C. LPO   D. RPO

21. A patient should be kept NPO prior to a cardiac catheterization for _____ hours.   21._____
    A. 2-4   B. 4-6   C. 8-12   D. 18-24

22. The _____ artery is the MOST commonly used site for arterial access for interventional cardiology.   22._____
    A. femoral   B. brachial   C. radial   D. carotid

23.   23._____

   According to the above EKG, what type of pacemaker does this patient have?
   A. Temporary   B. Atrial
   C. Ventricular   D. Dual-chambered

24. Which artery is MOST beneficial to use for a cardiac catheterization for a patient with severe respiratory issues?   24._____
    A. Femoral   B. Carotid   C. Radial   D. Popliteal

25. Contrast agents can be injected into all of the following solutions EXCEPT   25._____
    A. D5W   B. Ringer's Solution
    C. Normal Saline   D. Heparin

KEY (CORRECT ANSWERS)

1. C
2. D
3. D
4. B
5. B

6. A
7. C
8. C
9. A
10. D

11. A
12. A
13. B
14. B
15. C

16. B
17. D
18. A
19. C
20. D

21. C
22. A
23. B
24. C
25. D

EXAMINATION SECTION
TEST 1

DIRECTIONS: Each question or incomplete statement is followed by several suggested answers or completions. Select the one that BEST answers the question or completes the statement. *PRINT THE LETTER OF THE CORRECT ANSWER IN THE SPACE AT THE RIGHT.*

1. Each of the following is a parameter that should be considered when choosing an appropriate guidewire EXCEPT

    A. length   B. core   C. sheath   D. caliber

2. Discussing patient information with a friend outside the medical setting is a violation of the legal principle of

    A. slander
    C. assault
    B. professional negligence
    D. invasion of privacy

3. Of the following types of intensifying screens, which would produce the HIGHEST resolution images?

    A. High speed rare earth
    B. Molybdenum
    C. High speed calcium tungstate
    D. Slow calcium tungstate

4. Each of the following is a potential side effect of the coronary injection of iodine-containing contrast agents EXCEPT

    A. myocardial ischemia
    B. shortening QT interval
    C. cumulative renal toxicity
    D. T-wave inversion

5. During cardiopulmonary resuscitation involving one rescuer, compressions to the subject's heart are applied directly with the

    A. open palm
    C. heel of the hand
    B. flats of the fingertips
    D. closed fist

6. The average normal adult blood pressure is

    A. 120/40   B. 120/80   C. 100/60   D. 80/60

7. A patient's radial pulse should be taken

    A. at the carotid artery
    B. at the base of the thumb
    C. inside and slightly below the elbow
    D. inside the upper arm

8. Before bleeding can be visualized angiographically, it must occur at a rate of _____ cc/min.

    A. 0.5   B. 1   C. 3   D. 7

9. The PRIMARY ultrasound imaging method for the heart is

    A. chest roentgenography
    B. M-mode echocardiography
    C. Doppler echocardiography
    D. two-dimensional echocardiography

10. Each of the following is a material used in embolization EXCEPT

    A. Gianturco coil   B. coumadin
    C. bucrylate   D. gelfoam

11. Following removal of an arterial catheter, compression should be applied for AT LEAST _____ minutes.

    A. 5   B. 10   C. 30   D. 60

12. Which of the following radiographic projections will generally offer the BEST view for the left main coronary artery?

    A. 10° RAO   B. 20°-30° cranial
    C. 45° LAO/30° caudal   D. 45° LAO/20° cranial

13. Which of the following procedures will typically require the LOWEST single dosage of intravascular contrast media?

    A. Hepatic arteriography   B. Coronary angiography
    C. Abdominal aortography   D. Pulmonary arteriography

14. If used to prevent catheter thrombosis, how many units of heparin should be added for every cc of flush solution?

    A. 2-4   B. 50-100   C. 2,000   D. 5,000

15. The normal number of adult respirations per minute is

    A. 6-10   B. 12-16   C. 18-25   D. 20-30

16. Following the injection of contrast media, each of the following responses should be noted in the patient's medical chart EXCEPT

    A. flushed feeling immediately following injection
    B. mild dizziness following injection
    C. pain at puncture site
    D. mild itching following injection

17. The film sequence *2/sec x 3 sec: 1/sec x 4 sec: 2 delays* would MOST likely be used for

    A. splenic (portal vein) arteriography
    B. coronary angiography
    C. abdominal aortography
    D. inferior venocavography

18. Currently, the MAIN disadvantage associated with digital angiographic imaging is   18.____

    A. expensive technology
    B. poor contrast enhancement
    C. more invasive catheterization
    D. unwieldy image archiving and retrieval

19. In order to visualize the lymph nodes, _____ hour delayed film would be MOST useful.   19.____

    A. 1-2   B. 4-8   C. 14-18   D. 24-48

20. Which of the following medications is NOT involved in the management of a major anaphylactoid reaction to contrast agents?   20.____

    A. Hydrocortisone   B. Ephedrine
    C. Epinephrine   D. Cimetidine

21. The innermost wall of an artery is called the   21.____

    A. pith   B. intima
    C. adventitia   D. core

22. The MAIN advantage associated with the use of cut film changers, as opposed to the roll film type, is   22.____

    A. easier unloading
    B. faster film frequency
    C. higher film capacity
    D. better film-screen contact

23. Which of the following steps in the placement of a Greenfield vena cava filter would be performed FIRST?   23.____

    A. Inner dilator and guidewire are withdrawn
    B. Sheath is flushed with heparinized saline
    C. Incision site widened to 3-4 mm
    D. Filter capsule is positioned at release site

24. The injection time for 12 ml of intravascular contrast media, delivered at 2.5 ml/sec, would be _____ seconds.   24.____

    A. 0.5   B. 1.6   C. 2.7   D. 4.8

25. Stenosis is a term used to describe   25.____

    A. the separation of layers of a vascular structure
    B. the narrowing of a valve
    C. increased vascular pressure
    D. decreased vascular flow

KEY (CORRECT ANSWERS)

1. C
2. D
3. D
4. B
5. C

6. B
7. B
8. A
9. D
10. B

11. B
12. A
13. B
14. A
15. B

16. A
17. C
18. D
19. D
20. B

21. B
22. A
23. C
24. D
25. B

TEST 2

DIRECTIONS: Each question or incomplete statement is followed by several suggested answers or completions. Select the one that BEST answers the question or completes the statement. *PRINT THE LETTER OF THE CORRECT ANSWER IN THE SPACE AT THE RIGHT.*

1. Which of the following is a dimeric low-osmolarity contrast agent used in angiographic applications? 1.____

   A. Isovue
   B. Omnipaque
   C. Conray
   D. Hexabrix

2. During iliac angioplasty, the balloon is initially inflated for a period of 2.____

   A. 5 seconds
   B. 45 seconds
   C. 2 minutes
   D. 5 minutes

3. The pooling of blood due to arterial resistance failure is likely to cause _____ shock. 3.____

   A. hypoglycemic
   B. hypothermal
   C. neurogenic
   D. anaphylactic

4. The MAIN disadvantage associated with the use of Teflon catheters is 4.____

   A. low fluoroscopic visibility
   B. lack of friction
   C. low torque control
   D. stiffness

5. In ECG applications, what is the normal QRS duration (seconds) in adult patients? 5.____

   A. .01-.07
   B. .07-.10
   C. .12-.20
   D. .20-.32

6. For 2X magnification images, the MAXIMUM acceptable focal spot size is _____ mm. 6.____

   A. 0.3
   B. 1.0
   C. 1.7
   D. 3.0

7. A patient's heart rate should be measured by multiplying an irregular arrhythmia by 10 after counter the number of R waves that occur in _____ seconds. 7.____

   A. 3
   B. 6
   C. 30
   D. 60

8. For a pelvic and leg arteriogram, the catheter should be positioned _____ cm above the aortic bifurcation. 8.____

   A. 1
   B. 4
   C. 6
   D. 10

9. Which of the following catheter configurations is BEST suited for innominate and subclavian artery catheterization? 9.____

   A. Headhunter
   B. RIM
   C. RH
   D. S2

10. Each of the following are associated with the use of contrast agents that can be virtually eliminated with the use of low-osmolarity agents EXCEPT 10.____

A. nausea
C. renal toxicity
B. myocardial function
D. bradycardia

Questions 11-25.

DIRECTIONS: Questions 11 through 25 refer to the figure below, a diagram of the dorsocaudal surface of the heart. Place the letter that corresponds to each blood vessel or component in the space at the right.

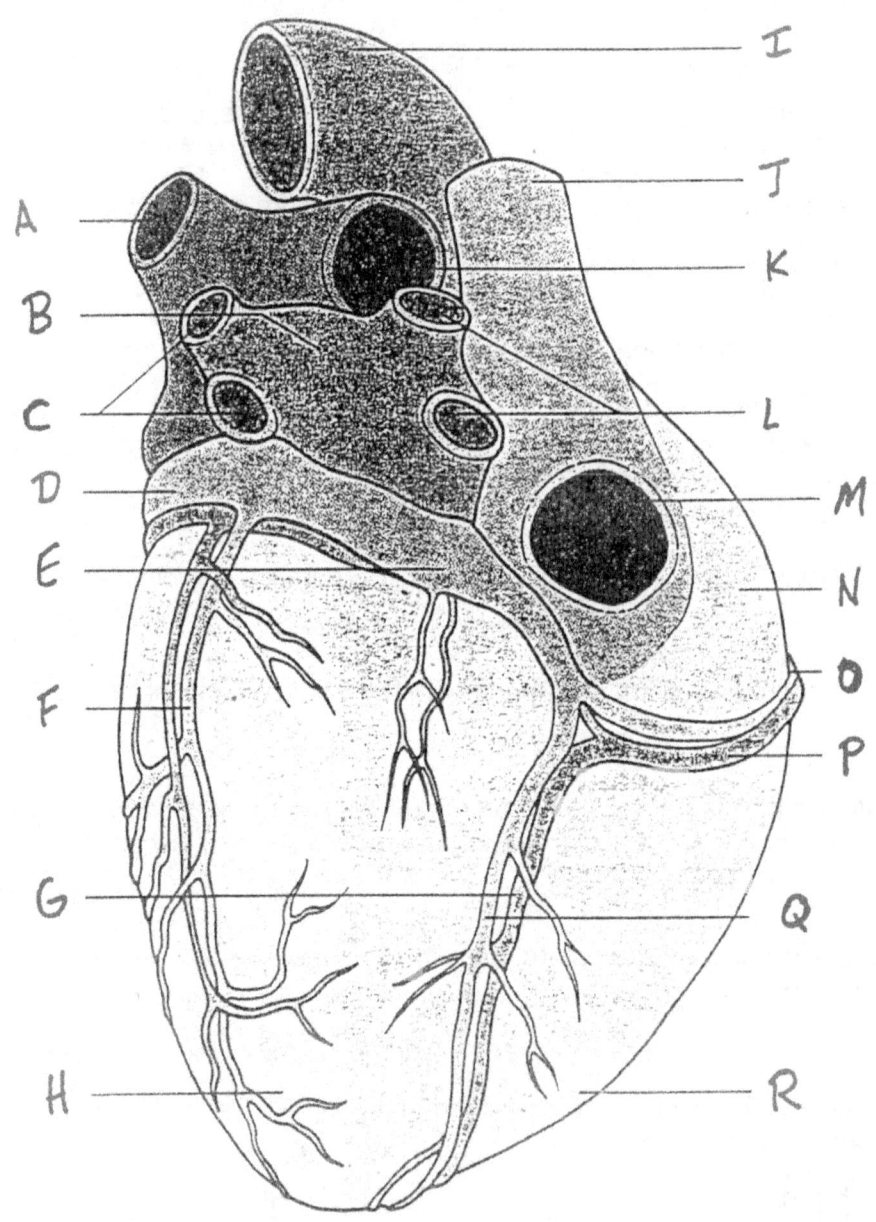

11. Posterior vein of left ventricle   11._____
12. Small cardiac vein   12._____
13. Coronary sinus   13._____
14. Left pulmonary artery   14._____
15. Right coronary artery   15._____
16. Great cardiac vein   16._____
17. Aorta   17._____
18. Posterior descending branch of right coronary artery   18._____
19. Left pulmonary veins   19._____
20. Inferior vena cava   20._____
21. Middle cardiac vein   21._____
22. Right pulmonary artery   22._____
23. Right pulmonary veins   23._____
24. Right atrium   24._____
25. Superior vena cava   25._____

KEY (CORRECT ANSWERS)

1. D   11. F
2. B   12. O
3. C   13. E
4. D   14. A
5. B   15. P

6. A   16. D
7. B   17. I
8. B   18. G
9. A   19. C
10. C   20. M

21. Q
22. K
23. L
24. N
25. J

TEST 3

DIRECTIONS: Each question or incomplete statement is followed by several suggested answers or completions. Select the one that BEST answers the question or completes the statement. *PRINT THE LETTER OF THE CORRECT ANSWER IN THE SPACE AT THE RIGHT.*

Questions 1-11.

DIRECTIONS: Questions 1 through 11 refer to the figure below, a diagram of the abdominal vasculature. Place the letter that corresponds to each blood vessel or component in the space at the right.

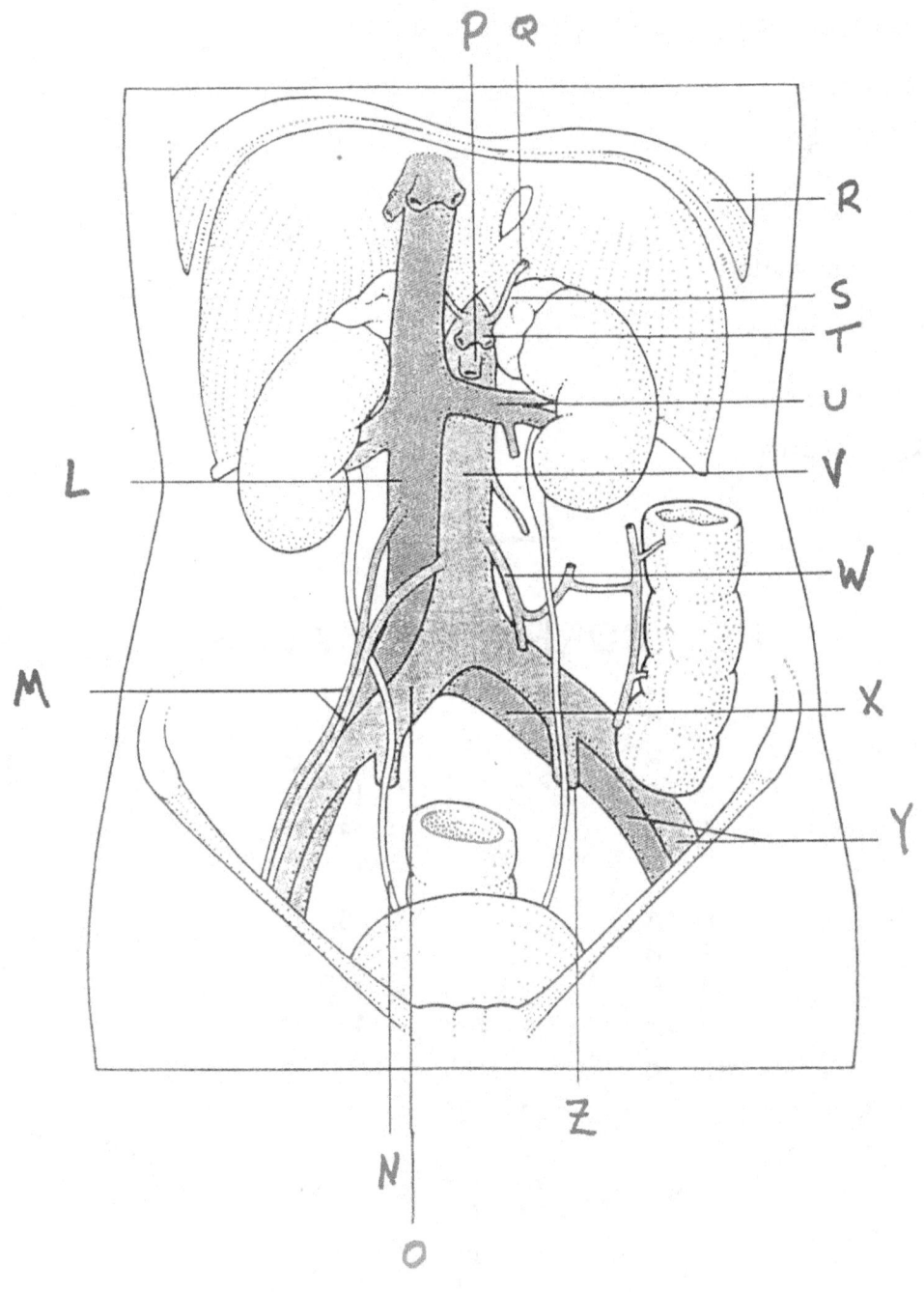

24

1. Celiac trunk
2. Inferior vena cava
3. Right common iliac artery
4. Abdominal aorta
5. External iliac artery and vein
6. Left crus
7. Gonadal artery and vein
8. Superior mesenteric artery
9. Left renal vein
10. Inferior mesenteric artery
11. Internal iliac artery

12. The chamber of the heart that is located MOST posteriorly is the
    A. left ventricle
    B. right ventricle
    C. right atrium
    D. left atrium

13. The PROPER patient position for a translumbar aortogram is
    A. LPO   B. RPO   C. supine   D. prone

14. The approximate total run time for a pulmonary arterio-gram is _____ seconds.
    A. 2   B. 4   C. 6   D. 10

15. During a biliary drainage procedure, a guidewire cannot be advanced beyond the obstruction.
    The catheter
    A. should be removed, while keeping the guidewire in place
    B. and guidewire should be removed and the procedure terminated
    C. should be left in place for internal drainage
    D. should be left in place for external drainage

16. Which of the following is NOT a contraindication for pulmonary digital subtraction angiography?
    A. Inability to suppress cough reflex
    B. Small lung capacity
    C. Dyspneia
    D. Low cardiac output

17. A patient has severe aortic stenosis.
    What modification should be made for the purpose of a left ventricular volume study?
    A. Decrease the injection time
    B. Decrease the injection rate

C. Use a laser-tipped catheter
D. Increase the catheter caliber

18. There are three distinct patterns of abnormal P waves during the sinus rhythm of an ECG.
    Which of the following is NOT one of these patterns?

    A. Right atrial enlargement
    B. Left atrial abnormality
    C. Biventricular hypertrophy
    D. P pulmonate

19. For a renal arteriogram, which of the following single dosages (ml) of contrast material would be within the recommended procedural average?

    A. 10   B. 20   C. 40   D. 60

20. Which of the following radiographic projections would typically be used to view the proximal right coronary artery?

    A. 30° RAO   B. 20°-30° cranial
    C. 30° LAO   D. 45° LAO/20° cranial

21. The MOST common complication associated with a transephatic catheterization is

    A. sepsis   B. hemothorax
    C. jaundice   D. hemorrhage

22. Which of the following devices provides a patient with the HIGHEST concentration of oxygen?

    A. Nonrebreathing mask   B. Venturi mask
    C. Aerosol mask   D. Enclosed tent

23. The needle gauge MOST appropriate for intraperitoneal biopsies is

    A. 12   B. 18   C. 22   D. 28

24. Which of the following types of angiographic catheters is MOST widely used?

    A. Polyethylene   B. Nylon
    C. Polyurethane   D. Teflon

25. In digital subtraction angiography, each of the following is possible EXCEPT

    A. electronic magnification
    B. conversion to analog imaging
    C. window adjustments
    D. pixel shifting

KEY (CORRECT ANSWERS)

1. T
2. L
3. O
4. V
5. Y

6. S
7. M
8. P
9. U
10. W

11. Z
12. D
13. D
14. C
15. D

16. B
17. B
18. C
19. A
20. C

21. A
22. A
23. C
24. A
25. B

TEST 4

DIRECTIONS: Each question or incomplete statement is followed by several suggested answers or completions. Select tne one that BEST answers the question or completes the statement. *PRINT THE LETTER OF THE CORRECT ANSWER IN THE SPACE AT THE RIGHT.*

Questions 1-8.

DIRECTIONS: Questions 1 through 8 refer to the figure below, a frontal diagram of the arteries associated with the subclavian area. Place the letter that corresponds to each blood vessel or component in the space at the right.

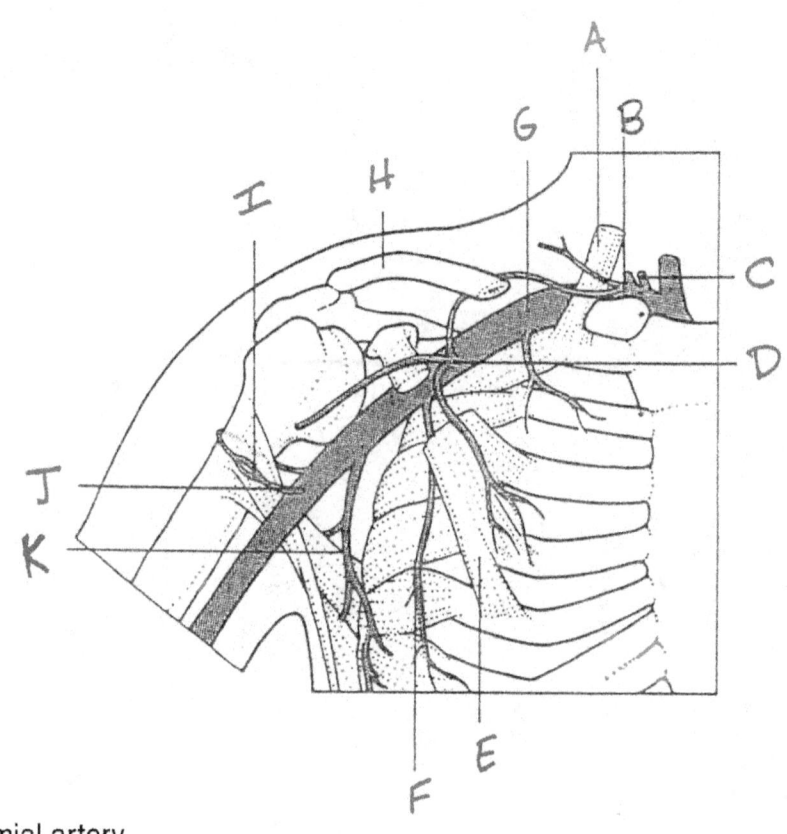

1. Thoracoacromial artery 1.___

2. Lateral pectoral artery 2.___

3. Axillary artery 3.___

4. Thyrocervical trunk 4.___

5. Anterior and posterior circumflex humeral arteries 5.___

6. Vertebral artery 6.___

7. Subscapular artery 7.___

8. Subclavian artery 8.___

9. The x-ray generator used for digital angiography typically is capable of _____ kVp at 1 mA, for rates up to 30 pulses per second.

   A. 25-35   B. 40-80   C. 60-120   D. 100-200

10. Each of the following could be a site for renal vein renin sampling EXCEPT

   A. inferior vena cava superior to renal veins
   B. main right renal vein
   C. abdominal aorta superior to renal veins
   D. inferior vena cava inferior to renal veins

11. What is the approximate injection rate of contrast material (ml/sec) used for gastroduodenal arteriography?

   A. 4   B. 12-15   C. 15-20   D. 25

12. Each of the following is an important factor involved in choosing an appropriate contrast agent EXCEPT

   A. cost
   B. side effect profile
   C. sodium content
   D. opacification

13. Which of the following is a result of a successful dilation procedure?

   A. *Increased* lumen diameter
   B. *Increased* vascular pressure
   C. *Decreased* vascular flow
   D. *Decreased* opacification

14. An automatic roll film changer uses _____ intensifying screens.

   A. 2   B. 3   C. 4   D. 5

15. Each of the following devices is recommended for intravascular foreign body retrieval EXCEPT

   A. snare loop catheter
   B. balloon tip retrieval catheter
   C. grasping device
   D. helical loop basket set

16. Which of the following is NOT a medication that would be involved in the pre-injection management of patients who have a history of previous adverse reaction to intravascular contrast agents?

   A. Ephedrine
   B. Atropine
   C. Hydrocortisone
   D. Benadryl

17. Which of the following right atrial A wave pressures (mm Hg) falls within the normal adult range?

   A. 6   B. 12   C. 18   D. 22

18. Embolization in angiographic applications may occur as a result of each of the following EXCEPT

    A. introduction of foreign material
    B. disruption of atheroma
    C. improper heparin dose
    D. catheter thrombosis

19. For peripheral arterial thrombolysis, an appropriate dosage of Urokinase would be 4,000 IU/min for a period of

    A. 30 minutes
    B. 2 hours
    C. 6 hours
    D. 12 hours

20. Each of the following is a segment of the middle cerebral artery EXCEPT

    A. horizontal
    B. pterygoid
    C. cortical
    D. sylvian

21. Which of the following is NOT an indication for percutaneous transephatic biliary drainage?

    A. Palliative decompression of malignant biliary obstruction
    B. Resting ischemia caused by stenosis
    C. Stone extraction
    D. Nonoperative management of fistulas

22. Each of the following is a possible cause of intestinal ischemia EXCEPT

    A. mesenteric vasoconstriction
    B. embolism
    C. renal toxicity
    D. thrombosis

23. Which of the following contrast material infusion rates is NOT used during a Whitaker test?
    _____ ml/min for 10 minutes.

    A. 5
    B. 10
    C. 15
    D. 20

24. Of the 12 standard ECG leads, which of the following is semidirect and unipolar?

    A. I
    B. V5
    C. aVL
    D. aVR

25. The bifurcation of the abdominal aorta forms the

    A. superior and inferior mesenteric arteries
    B. common iliacs
    C. carotids
    D. external iliacs

KEY (CORRECT ANSWERS)

1.	D	11.	A
2.	F	12.	C
3.	J	13.	A
4.	B	14.	A
5.	I	15.	C
6.	C	16.	B
7.	K	17.	A
8.	G	18.	C
9.	C	19.	B
10.	C	20.	B

21. B
22. C
23. D
24. B
25. B

EXAMINATION SECTION
TEST 1

DIRECTIONS: Each question or incomplete statement is followed by several suggested answers or completions. Select the one that BEST answers the question or completes the statement. *PRINT THE LETTER OF THE CORRECT ANSWER IN THE SPACE AT THE RIGHT.*

Questions 1-5.

DIRECTIONS: Questions 1 through 5 refer to the figure below, a diagram of several miscellaneous catheter configurations. Place the letter that corresponds to each configuration in the space at the right.

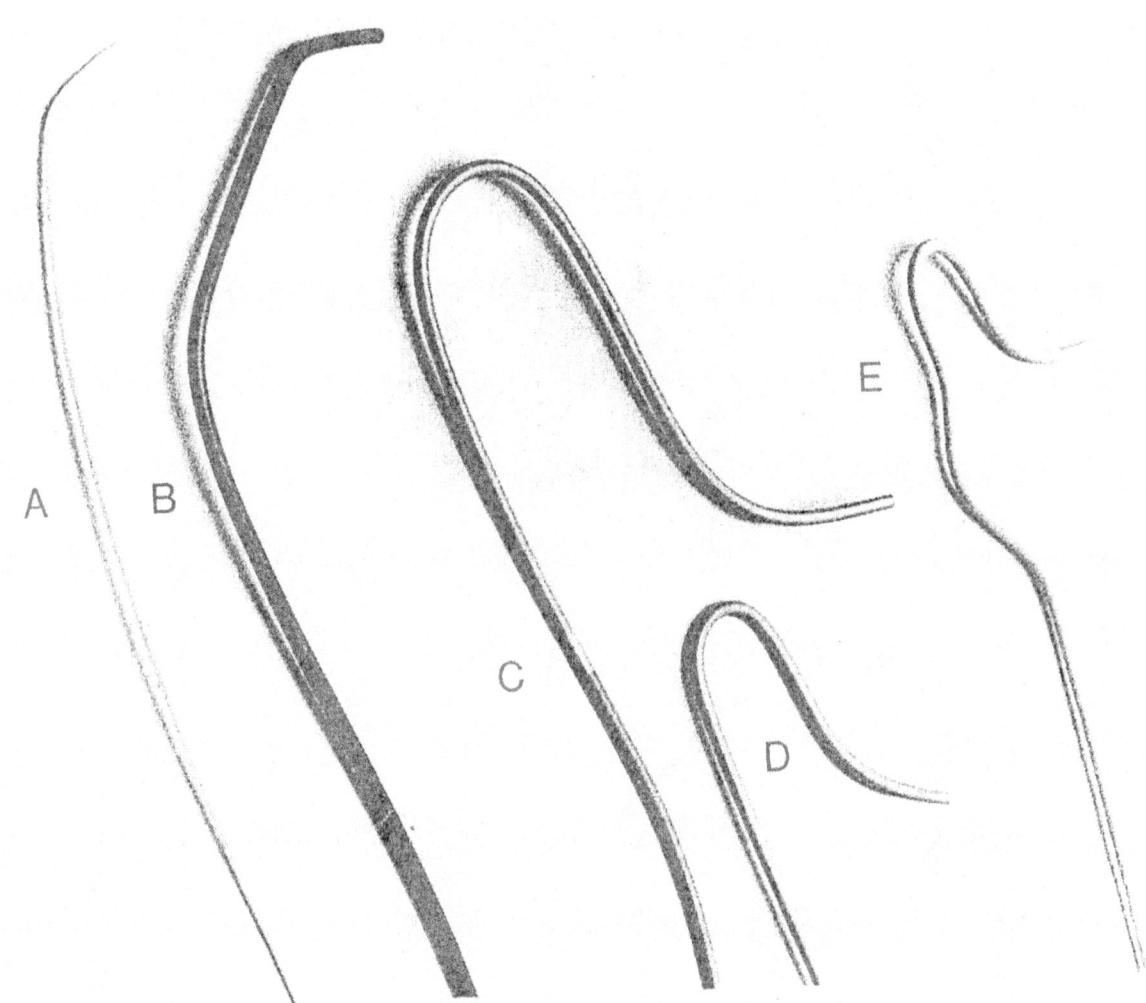

1. S2

2. S1

3. JB-1

4. H1

5. Mikaelsson

6. A patient's femoral pulse should be taken

   A. at the groin
   B. at the ankle
   C. just above and inside the knee
   D. just above and inside the ankle

7. A thoracic dissection that is classified as Type III

   A. originates in the ascending aorta and extends into the aortic arch, and for a variable distance beyond
   B. originates distal to the left subclavian artery origin, with variable distal extension
   C. does not involve the aortic arch
   D. is confined to the aortic arch

8. For localization of the major adrenal arteries, which of the following procedures would be MOST useful?

   A. Aortogram
   B. Lymphangiogram
   C. Selective celiac arteriogram
   D. Splenic arteriogram

9. A patient's pulmonary artery pressure is 50 mm Hg. How would this patient be categorized?

   A. Normal
   B. Mildly hypertensive
   C. Moderately hypertensive
   D. Severely hypertensive

10. For a myelogram, contrast material is introduced into the

    A. conus medullaris
    B. subarachnoid space
    C. sagittal sinus
    D. subdural space

11. The left atrium and ventricle are separated by the _____ valve.

    A. mitral
    B. pulmonary
    C. semilunar
    D. tricuspid

12. The aortic arch is in the _____ plane.

    A. sagittal
    B. transverse
    C. coronal
    D. medial

13. The ejection fraction of an adult left ventricle generally falls within the range of _____ %.

    A. 20-40   B. 30-50   C. 60-80   D. 70-90

14. During percutaneous biliary stone removal, the MAJOR concern is

    A. bile extravasion
    B. ductal rupture
    C. peritonitis
    D. liver hemorrhage

15. The bifurcation of the popliteal artery forms the

    A. anterior and posterior tibial arteries
    B. fibular artery
    C. plantar arch
    D. perforating arteries

16. To produce a typical filming rate for portal vein visualization, films should be exposed for _____ seconds.

    A. 1-5   B. 10-15   C. 20-25   D. 30-40

17. Which of the following is the PRIMARY indication for fibrinolytic therapy?

    A. Arterial occlusions
    B. Arterial stenosis
    C. Cardiac arrhythmias
    D. Pulmonary hypertension

18. If the left femoral artery is obstructed, the NEXT choice as a puncture location for catheterization of the abdominal aorta would be the _____ artery.

    A. right femoral
    B. right axillary
    C. left axillary
    D. left brachial

19. Which of the following filming sequences would MOST likely be used for renal arteriography?

    A. 3/sec x 2 sec: 1/sec x 2 sec: 2 delays
    B. 1-2/sec x 5-10sec
    C. 2/sec x 2 sec: 1/sec x 3 sec: 4 delays
    D. cine

20. For arteriography of the arm, the BEST position is arm _____, palm _____.

    A. flexed; up
    B. flexed; down
    C. extended; up
    D. extended; down

21. During ECG monitoring, the amplitude of a normal P wave does NOT usually exceed _____ mV.

    A. .10   B. .25   C. .50   D. .70

22. Which of the following procedures would typically employ the HIGHEST injection rate of contrast material?

    A. Thoracic aortogram
    B. Celiac arteriogram
    C. Coronary angiogram
    D. Splenic arteriogram

23. A normal peak systolic systemic pressure in an artery would be _____ mm Hg.

    A. 10   B. 60   C. 100   D. 140

24. Which of the following is a risk associated with pulmonary arteriography?

    A. Tachycardia
    B. Right bundle branch block
    C. T wave inversion
    D. Endocardial stain

25. Each of the following parameters must be specified and programmed into the system prior to each angiographic run EXCEPT

   A. total volume of injection
   B. linear rate rise
   C. injection rate
   D. injection/filming delay time

KEY (CORRECT ANSWERS)

1. C
2. D
3. A
4. B
5. E

6. A
7. B
8. A
9. C
10. B

11. A
12. A
13. C
14. C
15. A

16. C
17. A
18. D
19. A
20. C

21. B
22. A
23. C
24. B
25. B

TEST 2

DIRECTIONS: Each question or incomplete statement is followed by several suggested answers or completions. Select the one that BEST answers the question or completes the statement. *PRINT THE LETTER OF THE CORRECT ANSWER IN THE SPACE AT THE RIGHT.*

1. The PRIMARY indication for coronary angiography is   1.____

   A. valvular pathology
   B. post-infarction angina
   C. coronary atherosclerosis
   D. ventricular arrhythmias

2. In an ECG, the relative refractive period is represented by the   2.____

   A. QT interval
   B. down slope of the T wave
   C. U wave
   D. P wave

3. Which of the following is NOT involved in the management of vasovagal reactions to contrast agents?   3.____

   A. Airway assessment
   B. Slow intravenous administration of atropine
   C. Trendelenburg position
   D. Repeat of IV injection if bradycardia persists

Questions 4-10.

DIRECTIONS: Questions 4 through 10 refer to the figure shown on the following page, a diagram of the neck and facial blood supply. Place the letter that corresponds to each blood vessel or component in the space at the right.

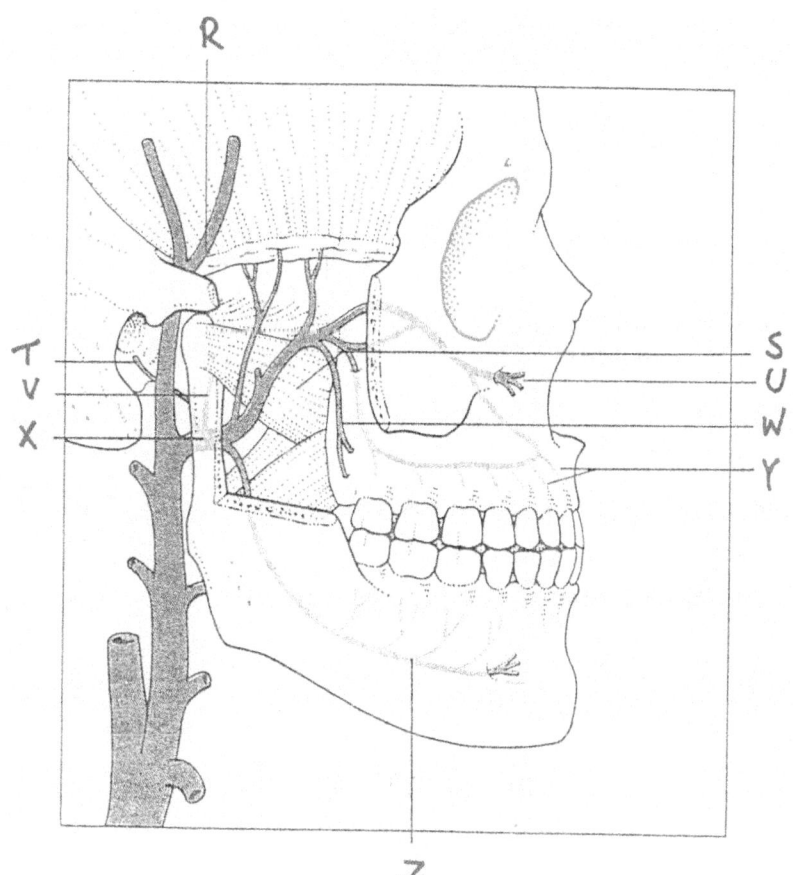

37

4. Inferior alveolar artery

5. Infra-orbital branches

6. Anterior tympanic artery

7. Maxillary artery

8. Posterior superior alveolar artery

9. Middle meningeal artery

10. Superficial temporal artery

11. Typically, non-ionic contrast agents must be heated to a temperature of _____ °C prior to injection through a standard diagnostic catheter.

    A. 19   B. 28   C. 37   D. 54

12. Typically, the balloon of an angioplasty catheter is filled with

    A. epinephrine
    B. contrast media and sterile saline
    C. contrast media *only*
    D. sterile saline solution *only*

13. For injecting the right heart with a single contrast material, a reasonable dose limit would be _____ cc.

    A. 3   B. 10   C. 35   D. 65

14. During cardiopulmonary resuscitation involving one rescuer, how many breaths are typically administered between sets of compressions?

    A. 2   B. 5   C. 10   D. 15

15. During a portal hypertension evaluation, a patient's CSP measurement is found to be 21. The patient

    A. is normal   B. has mild cirrhosis
    C. has moderate cirrhosis   D. has severe cirrhosis

16. During ECG monitoring, a normal T wave will always be upright in each of the following leads EXCEPT

    A. V_6 B. aV_R C. I   D. V_5

17. Which of the following is NOT a recommended criterion for exclusion from outpatient cardiac catheterization?

    A. Suspected left main coronary disease
    B. Renal disease
    C. Intercurrent febrile illness
    D. Uncontrolled systemic hypertension

18. Which of the following is an advantage associated with the use of roll film changers as opposed to the cut film type?

    A. Better storage of radiographs
    B. Easier loading
    C. Better film-screen contact
    D. Higher film capacity

19. During a lower limb venogram, films should be taken _____ seconds apart.

    A. 3-5　　　　B. 5-10　　　　C. 10-20　　　　D. 30-45

20. Typically, bradycardia is indicated by a heart rate _____ beats per minute.

    A. above 30　　B. above 50　　C. below 60　　D. below 120

21. Which of the following end diastolic volumes (ml/m^2) of the left ventricle falls within the normal adult range?

    A. 23　　　　B. 42　　　　C. 73　　　　D. 104

22. The 45° LAO/20° cranial radiographic projection is typically used to view each of the following arteries EXCEPT

    A. distal left main coronary
    B. horizontal left main coronary
    C. distal left main (coronary) bifurcation
    D. mid left anterior coronary, descending

23. Which of the following is NOT an indication for superior mesenteric arteriography?

    A. Gastrointestinal bleeding
    B. Vasculogenic impotence
    C. Arteriovenous malformation
    D. Intestinal ischemia from low flow

24. A lung mass casts a shadow that is 0.4 cm wide on a PA chest radiograph produced at 100 cm. The mass is located 6.2 cm from the film.
    What is the magnification factor?

    A. 0.90　　　B. 1.0　　　C. 1.07　　　D. 1.14

25. The border between the aortic bulb and the ascending aorta is known as the

    A. semilunar arch　　　　　B. supravalvular ring
    C. coronary cusp　　　　　　D. circle of Willis

KEY (CORRECT ANSWERS)

1. C
2. B
3. C
4. Z
5. U

6. T
7. X
8. W
9. V
10. R

11. C
12. B
13. B
14. A
15. D

16. B
17. C
18. D
19. B
20. C

21. C
22. D
23. B
24. C
25. B

TEST 3

DIRECTIONS: Each question or incomplete statement is followed by several suggested answers or completions. Select the one that BEST answers the question or completes the statement. *PRINT THE LETTER OF THE CORRECT ANSWER IN THE SPACE AT THE RIGHT.*

Questions 1-10.

DIRECTIONS: Questions 1 through 10 refer to the figure below, a diagram of the arteries of the pelvic wall. Place the letter that corresponds to each artery in the space at the right.

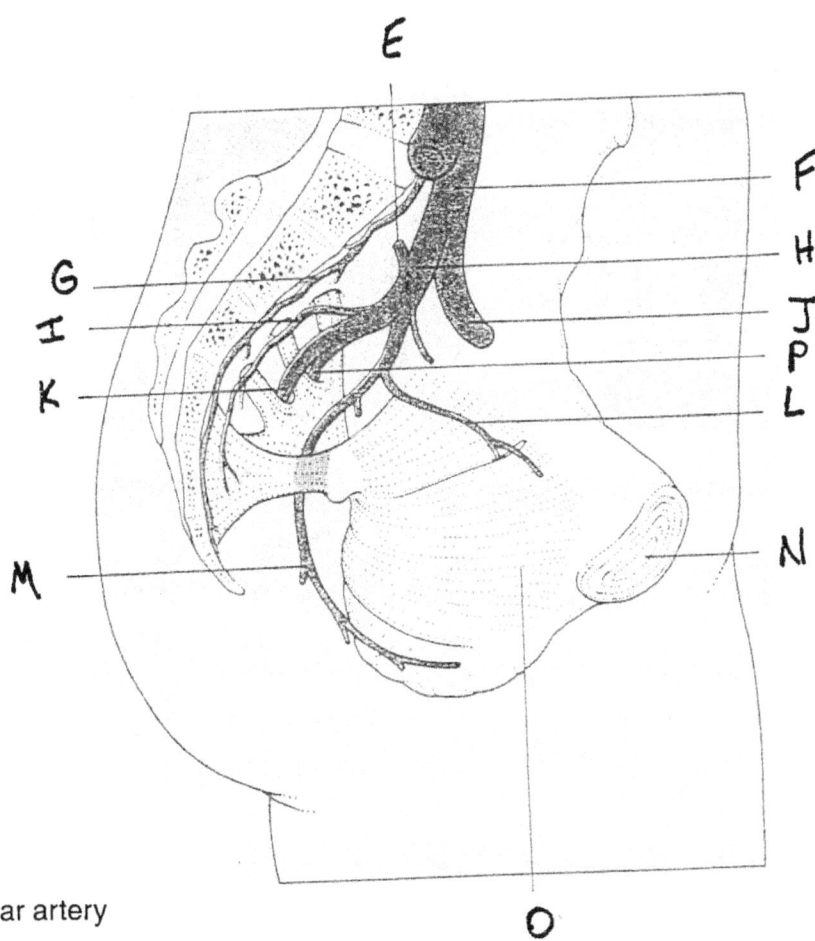

1. Iliolumbar artery   1._____
2. Obturator artery   2._____
3. Lateral sacral artery   3._____
4. Internal pudendal artery   4._____
5. External iliac artery   5._____
6. Superior gluteal artery   6._____
7. Median sacral artery   7._____
8. Internal iliac artery   8._____
9. Common iliac artery   9._____
10. Inferior gluteal artery   10._____

41

11. Customarily, catheterization images are filmed at a speed of _____ frames per second in left ventriculography.

    A. 15　　　B. 30　　　C. 60　　　D. 90

12. The first main branch of the subclavian artery is the _____ artery.

    A. basilar
    B. internal carotid
    C. brachiocephalic
    D. vertebral

13. Which of the following peak systolic pressure in the pulmonary artery (mm Hg) would be considered normal?

    A. 7　　　B. 12　　　C. 21　　　D. 40

14. For management of acute myocardial infarction, a PTCA procedure is combined with administration of

    A. antihistamine
    B. streptokinase
    C. epinephrine
    D. vasopressin

15. The time between exposure switch contact and the initiation of an exposure is known as _____ time.

    A. down　　　B. flex　　　C. phase-in　　　D. zero

16. What is the MOST commonly used embolization material?

    A. Detachable balloon
    B. Gianturco coil
    C. Polyvinyl alcohol
    D. Gelfoam

17. For coronary angiogram, which of the following single dosages (ml) of contrast material would be within the recommended procedural average?

    A. 5　　　B. 15　　　C. 25　　　D. 40

18. If used in angiographic applications, the usual intraarterial dose of nitroglycerin is _____ µg.

    A. 25　　　B. 50　　　C. 100　　　D. 250

19. For transluminal angioplasty, which of the following catheter configurations is MOST appropriate?

    A. Simmons
    B. Mikaelsson
    C. Curved tip
    D. Kensey

20. For angiography involving the right coronary artery, automatic pressure injectors should typically be preset at _____ ml/sec.

    A. 2-3　　　B. 3-4　　　C. 4-6　　　D. 5-7

21. Each of the following laboratory assessments would be indicated for an intravascular contrast study EXCEPT

    A. proteinuria
    B. albumin
    C. creatinine
    D. blood urea nitrogen

22. The brain is supplied directly by each of the following arteries EXCEPT   22.____

    A. left vertebral   B. left subclavian
    C. right carotid   D. left carotid

23. An abdominal aortogram demonstrates enlargement and opacification of branch arteries   23.____
    not typically seen in an aortogram.
    Which of the following is the MOST likely cause?

    A. Systolic-time injection
    B. Puncture of opposite arterial wall
    C. Aortic occlusion
    D. Too much contrast media

24. Which of the following represents the usual intra-arterial dosage of epinephrine used in   24.____
    angiographic applications?
    _____ mg diluted in _____ cc saline.

    A. .1; 500   B. .5; 500   C. 1; 1000   D. 5; 1000

25. Each of the following is a cause of *damping* during coronary catheterization EXCEPT   25.____

    A. ostial spasm around the catheter tip
    B. subselective engagement of the conus branch
    C. true ostial stenosis
    D. larger caliber of vessel

KEY (CORRECT ANSWERS)

1.	E	11.	C
2.	L	12.	D
3.	I	13.	C
4.	M	14.	B
5.	J	15.	C
6.	P	16.	D
7.	G	17.	A
8.	H	18.	C
9.	F	19.	D
10.	K	20.	A

21.	B
22.	B
23.	C
24.	B
25.	D

TEST 4

DIRECTIONS: Each question or incomplete statement is followed by several suggested answers or completions. Select the one that BEST answers the question or completes the statement. *PRINT THE LETTER OF THE CORRECT ANSWER IN THE SPACE AT THE RIGHT.*

1. The purpose of applying heparin to a wrapped wire is to

    A. ensure complete puncture
    B. reduce friction
    C. reduce unraveling
    D. reduce clotting

2. For coronary angiography, the catheter configuration MOST often used is the _____ French end-hole design.

    A. 4   B. 5   C. 6   D. 7

3. For ventriculography, _____ inch intensifying screen is usually the BEST choice.

    A. 2 or 3   B. 4.5 or 5   C. 6 or 7   D. 9

4. For very small vessels, embolization is BEST carried out by using

    A. polyvinyl alcohol
    B. absolute ethanol
    C. Gianturco coils
    D. gelfoam

5. Which of the following is NOT a disadvantage associated with the use of low-osmolarity contrast agents?

    A. Expense
    B. Increased patient discomfort
    C. Greater likelihood of clotting
    D. Higher viscosity

Questions 6-15.

DIRECTIONS: Questions 6 through 15 refer to the figure shown on the following page, a diagram of the arteries of the upper limb. Place the letter that corresponds to each artery in the space at the right.

2 (#4)

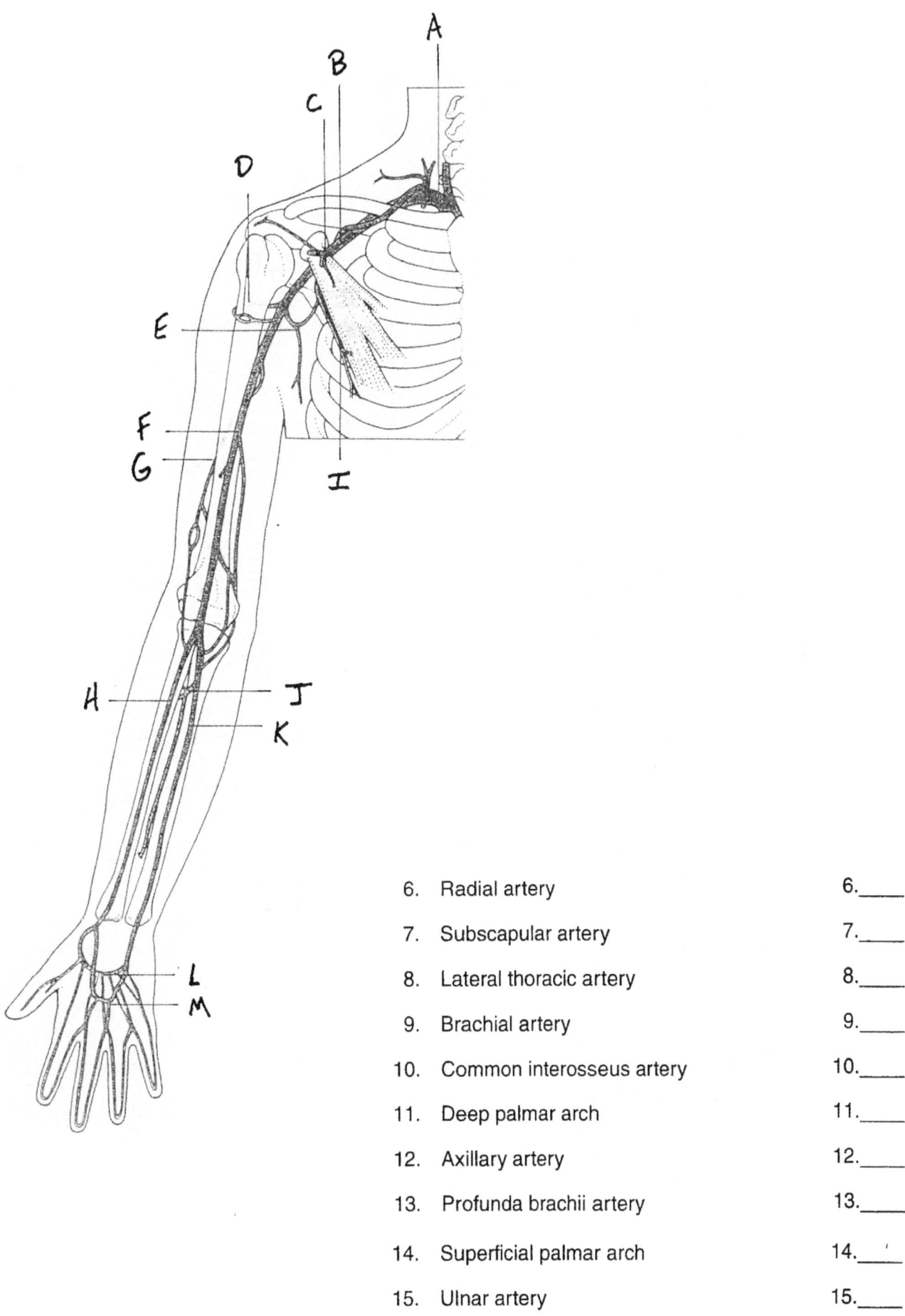

6. Radial artery 6.____
7. Subscapular artery 7.____
8. Lateral thoracic artery 8.____
9. Brachial artery 9.____
10. Common interosseus artery 10.____
11. Deep palmar arch 11.____
12. Axillary artery 12.____
13. Profunda brachii artery 13.____
14. Superficial palmar arch 14.____
15. Ulnar artery 15.____

16. The normal peak systolic pressure in the pulmonary artery is _____ mm Hg.

    A. 5-10   B. 20-30   C. 40-60   D. 100-120

17. For patients with cardiac conduction disorders that do not respond to medication, _____ is indicated.

    A. antibiotic treatments
    B. permanent pacemaker implantation
    C. PTCA procedures
    D. myelin therapy

18. The administration of diazepam is strongly contra-indicated by

    A. respiratory distress   B. nausea
    C. skin flush   D. nervous tension

19. A Whitaker test should be discontinued when/if the patient's renal pelvis pressure exceeds _____ cm of water.

    A. 22   B. 30   C. 40   D. 52

20. Vasovagal reactions to intravascular contrast agents are MOST often manifested by

    A. fibrillations
    B. hypertension and tachycardia
    C. nausea and dizziness
    D. hypotension and bradycardia

21. What type of catheter is used for lower extremity venography?

    A. Mikaelsson   B. Bentson
    C. 7 French   D. Butterfly needle

22. Which of the following rates for intravenous infusion (drops per minute) would MOST likely be considered safe?

    A. 5   B. 20   C. 40   D. 60

23. An endomyocardial biopsy is performed in the

    A. right atrium   B. right ventricle
    C. left atrium   D. left ventricle

24. For a selective vessel procedure involving an adult patient, the guide wire length will typically range from _____ cm.

    A. 20-40   B. 55-75   C. 100-150   D. 160-200

25. A patient has uretral blockage causing hydronephrosis. Which of the following procedures is indicated?

    A. Selective celiac arteriogram
    B. Nephrotic shunt
    C. Nephrostomy
    D. Percutaneous atherectomy

KEY (CORRECT ANSWERS)

1. D
2. D
3. D
4. B
5. B

6. H
7. E
8. I
9. F
10. J

11. L
12. B
13. G
14. M
15. K

16. B
17. B
18. A
19. C
20. D

21. D
22. B
23. B
24. C
25. C

EXAMINATION SECTION
TEST 1

DIRECTIONS: Each question or incomplete statement is followed by several suggested answers or completions. Select the one that BEST answers the question or completes the statement. *PRINT THE LETTER OF THE CORRECT ANSWER IN THE SPACE AT THE RIGHT.*

1. The PRIMARY risk associated with embolization procedures is

    A. reflux of steel coils
    B. migration of embolic materials
    C. bowel infarction
    D. reflux of gelfoam

    1._____

2. Which of the following catheter configurations is BEST suited for selective catheterization of small aortic branches that arise perpendicular to the aortic wall?

    A. JB-1   B. Pigtail
    C. RDP   D. Mikaelsson

    2._____

3. The MOST common indication for a femoral arteriogram is

    A. thrombosis
    B. arteriosclerotic obstructive lesions
    C. vascular fistula
    D. embolism

    3._____

4. For lymphangiography, what type of contrast media should be used? _____ compound.

    A. Oil-based dimeric   B. Water-soluble non-ionic
    C. Water-soluble ionic   D. Oil-based organic iodine

    4._____

5. Which of the following procedures will typically use the HIGHEST single dosage of intravascular contrast media?

    A. Splenic arteriography
    B. Coronary angiography
    C. Carotid cerebral arteriography
    D. Four-vessel cerebral arteriography

    5._____

6. For a selective renal angiogram, which of the following injection rates (ml/sec) would be ACCEPTABLE?

    A. 2   B. 9   C. 22   D. 32

    6._____

7. The MAIN indication for the infusion of a vasodilator is

    A. stenosis   B. occlusion
    C. vascular spasm   D. embolism

    7._____

8. Which of the following radiographic projections is NOT typically used to view the left circumflex coronary artery?

    A. 10°-20° RAO/20° caudal   B. 20°-30° cranial
    C. 40° LAO   D. 45° LAO/20° cranial

    8._____

49

9. The P wave of an ECG measures

   A. recovery
   B. ventricular depolarization
   C. atrial depolarization
   D. sinus rhythm

10. The film sequence *1/sec x 20 sec* would MOST likely be used for

    A. pulmonary arteriography
    B. splenic (portal vein) arteriography
    C. thoracic aortography
    D. gastroduodenal arteriography

11. Which of the following is NOT a factor predisposing a patient to myocardial infarction?

    A. Recent subendocardial infarction
    B. Unstable angina
    C. Cerebrovascular episodes
    D. Insulin-requiring diabetes

12. What is the approximate injection rate of contrast material (ml/sec) used for a hepatic arteriogram?

    A. 6-10   B. 12-15   C. 20   D. 35

13. What is the term for the outer layer of a vascular structure?

    A. Adventitia
    B. Intima
    C. Pith
    D. Cambium

14. The MOST commonly used entry site for pulmonary arteriography is the

    A. right brachial artery
    B. right common femoral vein
    C. left axillary artery
    D. right axillary artery

15. Each of the following is an example of a revascularization technique used to restore blood flow to an ischemic extremity EXCEPT

    A. angioplasty
    B. basket catheterization
    C. bypass grafting
    D. endarterectomy

16. The aorta and left ventricle are separated by the _____ valve.

    A. mitral   B. pulmonary   C. semilunar   D. tricuspid

17. The use of an arterial sheath during coronary arteriography may be contraindicated by

    A. quick catheter changes
    B. long catheterization duration
    C. pressure monitoring
    D. puncture site diameter

18. Which of the following is NOT an indication for placement of an inferior vena cava filter? 18._____

    A. Deep venous thrombosis
    B. Chronic pulmonary hypertension
    C. Dissecting aneurysm
    D. Recurrent pulmonary thromboembolism

19. Of the arteries of the leg, the _____ artery is MOST often occluded by embolisms. 19._____

    A. posterior tibial   B. superficial femoral
    C. descending genicular   D. popliteal

20. In ECG applications, what is the normal PR interval, in seconds, in adult patients? 20._____

    A. .01-.07   B. .07-.10   C. .12-.20   D. .20-.32

21. For the implantation of a permanent pacemaker, the _____ is the vessel typically used. 21._____

    A. jugular vein   B. subclavian artery
    C. brachial vein   D. subclavian vein

22. The MAIN disadvantage associated with the use of polyurethane catheters is 22._____

    A. difficult to reshape   B. low radio-opacity
    C. friction   D. low torque control

23. Each of the following is a risk associated with iliac angioplasty EXCEPT 23._____

    A. acute thrombosis
    B. occlusive arterial dissection
    C. renal artery spasm
    D. distal embolization

24. For a common carotid injection of contrast media, a reasonable dose limit would be _____ cc. 24._____

    A. 7   B. 10   C. 25   D. 50

25. A thoracic dissection that is classified as Type I 25._____

    A. originates in the ascending aorta and extends into the aortic arch, and for a variable distance beyond
    B. originates distal to the left subclavian artery origin, with variable distal extension
    C. does not involve the aortic arch
    D. is confined to the aortic arch

KEY (CORRECT ANSWERS)

1. B
2. D
3. B
4. D
5. D

6. B
7. C
8. B
9. C
10. B

11. C
12. A
13. A
14. B
15. B

16. C
17. D
18. C
19. B
20. C

21. D
22. C
23. C
24. C
25. A

TEST 2

DIRECTIONS: Each question or incomplete statement is followed by several suggested answers or completions. Select the one that BEST answers the question or completes the statement. *PRINT THE LETTER OF THE CORRECT ANSWER IN THE SPACE AT THE RIGHT.*

Questions 1-10.

DIRECTIONS: Questions 1 through 10 refer to the figure below, a frontal diagram of the lower limb's blood supply. Place the letter that corresponds to each artery in the space at the right.

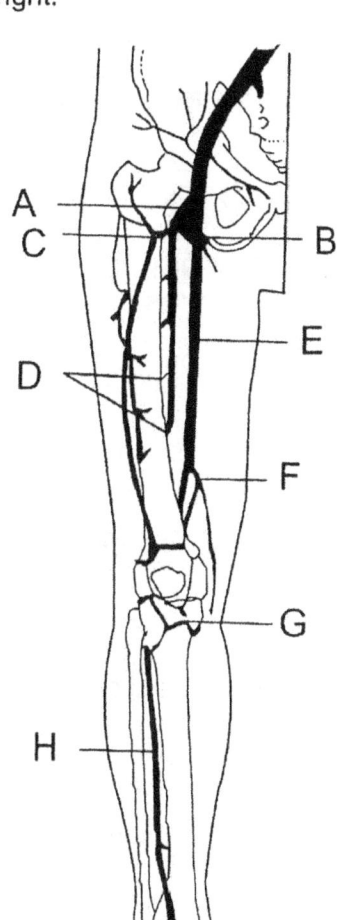

1. Dorsalis pedis artery
2. Perforating arteries
3. Descending genicular artery
4. Profunda femoris artery
5. Femoral artery
6. Anterior tibial artery
7. Anastomosis
8. Medial circumflex artery
9. Lateral circumflex artery
10. Arcuate artery

1.____
2.____
3.____
4.____
5.____
6.____
7.____
8.____
9.____
10.____

11. Which of the following medications is administered in order to control cardiac arrhythmias?

    A. Benadryl   B. Quinidine procainimide
    C. Heparin   D. Digitalis

12. Which of the following catheter configurations is BEST suited for a nephrostomy?

    A. Simmons with single end hole
    B. RIM
    C. Pigtail with multiple side holes
    D. RH

13. Which of the following steps in the insertion of a biliary endoprosthesis would be performed LAST?

    A. Endoprosthesis loaded onto stiffening cannula
    B. Contrast material injected
    C. Track dilated with high-pressure angioplasty balloon
    D. Internal-external catheter is removed

14. Minor allergic reactions to intravascular contrast agents typically include the following EXCEPT

    A. urticaria   B. sneezing
    C. vomiting   D. hypotension

15. To increase deep vein filling during leg venography, tourniquets should be applied at

    A. mid-thigh and mid-calf   B. mid-calf and ankle
    C. mid-thigh and knee   D. the knee and ankle

16. The addition of side holes in a catheter will typically produce an approximate increase in the total flow rate of _____ %.

    A. 5   B. 15   C. 40   D. 65

17. Which of the following patient positions is assumed for a Whitaker test?

    A. Lateral   B. Oblique   C. Prone   D. Supine

18. MOST commonly, the narrowing of the renal artery is caused by

    A. fused kidneys   B. stenosis
    C. stone occlusion   D. arteriosclerosis

19. In thoracic aortography, the catheter should always be positioned just above the _____ valve.

    A. mitral   B. pulmonary   C. semilunar   D. tricuspid

20. Which of the following is typically used to control gastrointestinal bleeding?

    A. Tolazoline   B. Vasopressin
    C. Epinephrine   D. Heparin

21. A normal mean brachial artery pressure would be _____ mm Hg.

    A. 10 B. 60 C. 90 D. 150

22. A multiple side hole catheter would typically be used in angiographic imaging involving the

    A. renal artery
    C. mesenteric region
    B. abdominal aorta
    D. cerebrum

23. For a thoracic aortogram, which of the following single dosages, in ml, of contrast material would be within the recommended procedural average?

    A. 10 B. 20 C. 30 D. 60

24. Each of the following is effective in reducing scatter during biplane angiography EXCEPT

    A. air-gap magnification
    B. exposure alternation
    C. horizontal cross-hatch grid
    D. vertical cross-hatch grid

25. Which of the following filming sequences would MOST likely be used for renal and inferior venocavogram?

    A. 2/sec x 2 sec: 1/sec x 2 sec
    B. 1-2/sec x 5-10 sec
    C. 2/sec x 4-8 sec
    D. cine

4 (#2)

KEY (CORRECT ANSWERS)

1.	J		11.	B
2.	D		12.	C
3.	F		13.	B
4.	A		14.	D
5.	E		15.	D
6.	H		16.	B
7.	G		17.	C
8.	B		18.	D
9.	C		19.	C
10.	I		20.	B

21. C
22. B
23. D
24. C
25. C

TEST 3

DIRECTIONS: Each question or incomplete statement is followed by several suggested answers or completions. Select the one that BEST answers the question or completes the statement. *PRINT THE LETTER OF THE CORRECT ANSWER IN THE SPACE AT THE RIGHT.*

1. A pulmonary embolism is MOST accurately demonstrated by

   A. CT of the chest
   B. AP and lateral chest radiographs
   C. a cardiac angiogram
   D. a pulmonary arteriogram

2. Which of the following is NOT a typical risk involved in fibrinolytic therapy?

   A. Remote-site bleeding
   B. Arterial dissection
   C. Dislodgement of central thrombi
   D. Peripheral embolization

3. Each of the following is used as an embolic medium in angiographic applications EXCEPT

   A. barium sulfate
   B. silicon elastomer
   C. balloon catheters
   D. microfibrillar sponges

4. Which of the following projections is BEST for filming the biliary ductal system?

   A. AP   B. Lateral   C. RPO   D. 15 LAO

5. Which of the following is a non-ionic contrast agent?

   A. Hypaque   B. Hexabrix   C. Isopaque   D. Optiray

6. Each of the following procedures is involved in the Seldinger technique EXCEPT

   A. surgically opening the artery
   B. removing the guide wire
   C. piercing the artery completely with a compound needle
   D. introduction of a guide wire through the compound needle

7. Which of the following coronary branches lies in the atrio-ventricular plane?

   A. Circumflex
   B. Posterior descending
   C. Diagonal
   D. Obtuse marginal

8. The common iliacs join to form the

   A. superior mesenteric artery
   B. abdominal aorta
   C. inferior vena cava
   D. superior vena cava

9. The brachial approach for arteriography is often preferred for each of the following types of patients EXCEPT

   A. patients with diminished radial pulse
   B. obese patients
   C. patients with wide pulse pressure
   D. patients with peripheral vascular disease

10. Each of the following is an ECG manifestation of right ventricular hypertrophy EXCEPT

   A. typical RVH pattern with anterior and rightward displacement of the main QRS vector
   B. posterior and rightward displacement of the main QRS axis
   C. incomplete right bundle branch block
   D. widening of the QRS/T angle

11. Each of the following is a recommended criterion for exclusion of a patient from outpatient cardiac catheterization EXCEPT

   A. anticoagulant therapy
   B. renal insufficiency
   C. unstable angina
   D. age greater than 70 years

12. What is the term for a drop in diastolic pressure?

   A. Depolarization
   B. Ventricularization
   C. Inversion
   D. Asystole

13. Currently, digital subtraction angiography is MOST useful for

   A. lymphangiography
   B. lower limb venography
   C. pulmonary angiography
   D. thoracic aortography

14. In most catheterization laboratories, the maximal pressure cutoff for ventriculography is _____ psi.

   A. 500   B. 750   C. 1000   D. 1500

15. A patient is experiencing esophageal varicaeal bleeding. Which of the following vessels should be catheterized?

   A. Left gastric artery
   B. Superior mesenteric artery
   C. Coronary gastric veins
   D. Inferior mesenteric artery

16. The right _____ arteries do NOT pass posterior to the inferior vena cava.

   A. lumbar
   B. gonadal
   C. renal
   D. middle suprarenal

17. Which of the following catheter configurations is used PRIMARILY for injection of large vessels with relatively high flow rates?

   A. JB-1   B. Pigtail   C. CI   D. S2

18. Which of the following is part of an automatic film changer compression table?

    A. Radiographic film
    B. Lens
    C. Grid
    D. Intensifying screens

19. Each of the following is an ECG criterion for the diagnosis of left anterior hemiblock EXCEPT

    A. direction of the main QRS axis in the frontal plane from about -45° to -85°
    B. Q wave in the III lead
    C. initial QRS vector directed to the right and anteriorly
    D. QRS duration less than .12 second

20. Which of the following procedures involves a direct puncture of the aorta?

    A. Splenic arteriography
    B. Percutaneous catheter aortography
    C. Translumbar aortography
    D. Superior mesenteric arteriography

21. Endocardial staining is a possible complication of

    A. ventriculography
    B. coronary angiography
    C. thoracic aortography
    D. the Whitaker test

22. The opthalmic artery branches from the _____ artery.

    A. basilar
    B. internal carotid
    C. vertebral
    D. maxillary

23. Which of the following is NOT among the most widely used ionic contrast agents?

    A. Angiovist   B. Isopaque   C. Hypaque   D. Renografin

24. For a hepatic wedge study, the _____ is injected with contrast media.

    A. abdominal aorta
    B. portal vein
    C. superior mesenteric artery
    D. splenic vein

25. Which of the following angiographic applications would typically require the contrast material of HIGHEST concentration?

    A. Venogram
    B. Percutaneous transephatic cholangiogram
    C. Aortic arch
    D. Renal artery

KEY (CORRECT ANSWERS)

1.	D	11.	B
2.	B	12.	B
3.	A	13.	C
4.	A	14.	C
5.	D	15.	C
6.	A	16.	B
7.	A	17.	B
8.	C	18.	D
9.	A	19.	B
10.	D	20.	C

21. A
22. B
23. B
24. B
25. C

TEST 4

DIRECTIONS: Each question or incomplete statement is followed by several suggested answers or completions. Select the one that BEST answers the question or completes the statement. *PRINT THE LETTER OF THE CORRECT ANSWER IN THE SPACE AT THE RIGHT.*

1. For visualizing the superior vena cava, a catheter should be placed in the

    A. pulmonary vein
    B. axillary or subclavian vein
    C. aortic arch
    D. superior portion of the superior vena cava

2. For calculating magnification, the PROPER formula is

    A. OFD/FOD (SOD/OID)
    B. FFD/FOD (SID/SOD)
    C. FOD/FFD (SOD/SID)
    D. FFD/OFD (OID/SID)

3. During cardiopulmonary resuscitation involving one rescuer, how many compressions are typically administered between sets of breaths?

    A. 2   B. 5   C. G. 10   D. 15

4. Each of the following is an immediate hemodynamic effect associated with contrast material injected for ventriculo-graphy EXCEPT

    A. vasoconstriction
    B. reflex increase in heart rate
    C. slight drop in systemic arterial pressure
    D. transient depression of left ventricular contractility

5. Which of the following is an acceptable placement of catheter side holes?

    A. At tapered tip
    B. Alternating opposite
    C. At curvature
    D. Directly opposite

6. Each adrenal gland is supplied by _____ arteries.

    A. 2   B. 3   C. 4   D. 5

7. When a severe, unexpected allergic reaction to a contrast agent occurs, the MOST common response is an IV administration of

    A. prednisone
    B. nifedipine
    C. cortisone
    D. epinephrine

8. Which of the following is included in angiographic post-procedural orders?

    A. Creatinine study
    B. PTT study
    C. Vital sign check
    D. BUN count

9. An object is placed 20" from the image receptor and 20" from the x-ray tube source. The magnification factor will be

    A. 1   B. 1.5   C. 2   D. 3

10. The muscular layer between the ventricles of the heart is the
    A. pericardium
    B. endocardium
    C. epicardium
    D. myocardium

11. What size balloon, in mm, is typically used for renal arterial angioplasty?
    A. 0.5
    B. 1
    C. 5
    D. 10

12. In order to reduce the possibility of post-puncture hematoma following an angioplasty,
    A. a smaller gauge of needle should be used
    B. the brachial approach should be used, rather than femoral
    C. the puncture site is dilated, rather than direct catheter insertion
    D. the puncture site should be more superior than previously

13. To reduce patient anxiety prior to catheterization, which of the following should be administered?
    A. Nifedipine
    B. Diazepam
    C. Atropine
    D. Nitroglycerin

14. For the kind of magnification required by special procedures such as PTCA, which type of intensifying screen is usually the BEST choice?
    A. 2 or 3 inch
    B. 4.5 or 5 inch
    C. 6 or 7 inch
    D. 9 inch

15. Which of the following catheter configurations is BEST suited for pulmonary arteriography?
    A. Simmons
    B. RIM
    C. Grollman
    D. Curved tip

16. Which of the following side effects, associated with the use of contrast agents, is only partially reduced by the use of low-osmolarity agents?
    A. Anaphylaxis
    B. Increased intravascular volume
    C. T-wave alterations
    D. Arterial vasodilation

17. The branch of the internal carotid artery with the LARGEST diameter is the _____ artery.
    A. posterior parietal
    B. posterior cerebral
    C. middle cerebral
    D. anterior cerebral

18. Typically, an IV is placed _____ inches above the venous point of entry.
    A. 6-10
    B. 12-18
    C. 18-24
    D. 36-48

19. Of the 12 standard ECG leads, which of the following is indirect and unipolar?
    A. I
    B. aV_L
    C. V_2
    D. III

3 (#4)

20. The descending sigmoid and rectal colon are supplied by the _____ artery.

    A. inferior mesenteric
    B. superior mesenteric
    C. ileocolic
    D. marginal

21. Which of the following lymph node groups is located in the pelvis?

    A. Anterior tibial
    B. Hypogastric
    C. Axillary
    D. Mesenteric

22. Each of the following is an advantage associated with the femoral approach in catheterization EXCEPT

    A. better for patients with aortic regurgitation
    B. can be performed repeatedly at intervals
    C. lower infection risk
    D. arterial repair not required

23. The PRIMARY indication for upper limb venography is

    A. trauma evaluation
    B. recovery of embolism
    C. evaluation of thrombosis
    D. evaluation of arteriovenous shunt

24. The FIRST major branch of the abdominal aorta is the

    A. portal vein
    B. celiac artery
    C. superior mesenteric artery
    D. hepatic artery

25. The *Cobra* catheter configuration is used for each of the following EXCEPT

    A. celiac arteriography
    B. thoracic aortography
    C. splenic arteriography
    D. hepatic arteriography

KEY (CORRECT ANSWERS)

1. B
2. B
3. D
4. C
5. B

6. B
7. D
8. C
9. C
10. D

11. C
12. C
13. B
14. B
15. C

16. A
17. C
18. C
19. B
20. A

21. B
22. A
23. C
24. B
25. B

EXAMINATION SECTION
TEST 1

DIRECTIONS: Each question or incomplete statement is followed by several suggested answers or completions. Select the one that BEST answers the question or completes the statement. *PRINT THE LETTER OF THE CORRECT ANSWER IN THE SPACE AT THE RIGHT.*

Questions 1-6.

DIRECTIONS: Questions 1 through 6 refer to the figure below, a diagram of blood vessels near the aortic arch. Place the letter that corresponds to each in the space at the right.

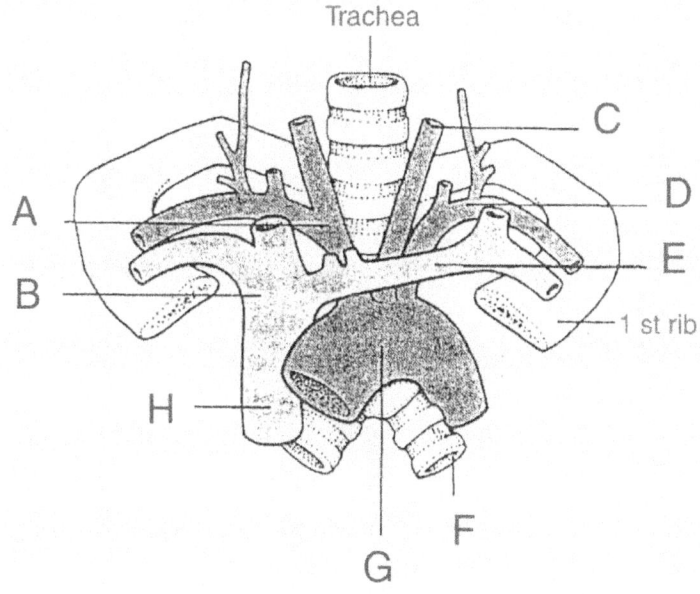

1. Right brachiocephalic vein   1.____

2. Left common carotid artery   2.____

3. Superior vena cava   3.____

4. Left subclavian artery   4.____

5. Brachiocephalic trunk   5.____

6. Left brachiocephalic vein   6.____

7. Which of the following is MOST commonly a symptom of a hypotensive reaction to cardiac catheterization?   7.____

   A. Nausea
   B. Brachial constriction
   C. Increased warmth of the skin
   D. Edema

65

8. To most accurately confirm hypertension, a _____ angiogram should be studied.

   A. renal B. coronary C. splenic D. cerebral

9. _____ mm film is commonly used for cine fluorography.

   A. 8 B. 12 C. 16 D. 24

10. Which of the following procedures would typically employ the LOWEST injection rate of contrast material?

    A. Abdominal aortogram
    B. Splenic arteriogram
    C. Superior venocavogram
    D. Inferior mesenteric arteriogram

11. What is the term for the separation of the walls of the aorta?

    A. Dissection B. Stenosis
    C. Intimation D. Embolism

12. A patient suffers myocardial ischemia during coronary angiography. The patient presents marked arterial hypertension and does not respond to an administration of nitroglycerin. The NEXT response should be to

    A. reverse heparin at the conclusion of the procedure
    B. administer sublingual nifedipine
    C. place an intra-aortic counterpulsation balloon in the contralateral femoral artery
    D. administer propranolol

13. For a pulmonary arteriogram, which of the following TOTAL doses, in ml, of contrast material would be within the recommended procedural average?

    A. 20 B. 80 C. 150 D. 225

14. The sylvian triangle is composed of the _____ artery and branches.

    A. middle cerebral B. carotid
    C. subclavian D. posterior communication

15. For lower extremity venography, the BEST insertion point is the

    A. plantar arch B. vein of the big toe
    C. great saphenous vein D. femoral vein

16. In order to obtain pulmonary arterial pressure measurements, a(n) _____ must be used.

    A. stethoscope B. transducer
    C. pigtail catheter D. Foley catheter

17. Which of the following coronary branches lies in the interventricular plane?

    A. Left anterior descending B. Conus
    C. Sinus node D. Right coronary

18. For the sterilization of electronic equipment, which method is acceptable? 18.____

    A. Pressurized steam B. Acetone
    C. Boiling D. Gas

19. Which of the following is NOT a risk associated with celiac arteriography? 19.____

    A. Arterial thrombosis B. Splenic infarction
    C. Colonic ischemia D. Gastric infarction

20. Customarily, catheterization images are filmed at a speed of _____ frames per second for coronary angiography. 20.____

    A. 15 B. 30 C. 60 D. 90

21. The MOST common indication for hepatic arteriography is 21.____

    A. hepatic arterial evaluation
    B. presurgical vascular mapping
    C. aneurysm evaluation
    D. embolization preparation

22. Most commonly, the Seldinger technique involves an approach through the _____ artery. 22.____

    A. brachial B. subclavian
    C. femoral D. superior mesenteric

23. For the insertion of a vena cava filter, a _____-inch guidewire is normally used. 23.____

    A. .015 B. .028 C. .035 D. .038

24. Which of the following is NOT used in roll film changers? 24.____

    A. Manual knife
    B. Supply and receiving magazine
    C. Automatic exposure control
    D. Program selector

25. Which patient position is BEST for the evaluation of the aortic arch? 25.____

    A. PA B. 35°-45° RPO
    C. Supine D. AP

KEY (CORRECT ANSWERS)

1. B
2. C
3. H
4. D
5. A

6. E
7. C
8. A
9. C
10. D

11. A
12. B
13. C
14. A
15. B

16. B
17. A
18. D
19. C
20. B

21. B
22. C
23. D
24. C
25. B

TEST 2

DIRECTIONS: Each question or incomplete statement is followed by several suggested answers or completions. Select the one that BEST answers the question or completes the statement. *PRINT THE LETTER OF THE CORRECT ANSWER IN THE SPACE AT THE RIGHT.*

1. Typically, anticoagulant medications should be withheld no later than _____ hours prior to angiography.   1.____

   A. 2   B. 4   C. 12   D. 24

2. End diastolic pressure minus end systolic pressure will yield the stroke volume of the   2.____

   A. right atrium   B. right ventricle
   C. left atrium   D. left ventricle

3. For displaying a magnified image of the central portion of the input phosphor, which type of intensifying screen is usually the BEST choice? _____ inch.   3.____

   A. 2 or 3   B. 4.5 or 5   C. 6 or 7   D. 9

4. _____ is NOT an indication for pulmonary arteriography.   4.____

   A. Pulmonary arteriovenous malformation
   B. Pulmonary hypertension
   C. Aneurysm evaluation
   D. Pulmonary embolism diagnosis

5. In a functional rhythm, a P wave appears   5.____

   A. upright and uniform   B. level
   C. irregularly downward   D. inverted

6. A nonselective injection of contrast media is made into the abdominal aorta, about 1-2 cm above the renal arteries. Which of the following would be LEAST likely to be visualized? _____ artery.   6.____

   A. Left suprarenal   B. Iliolumbar
   C. Inferior mesenteric   D. Right renal

7. Which of the following left atrial V wave pressures, in mm Hg, falls within the normal adult range?   7.____

   A. 1   B. 12   C. 25   D. 32

8. Each of the following is a type of vasodilator used in angiographic applications EXCEPT   8.____

   A. nifedipine   B. tolazaline
   C. vasopressin   D. nitroglycerin

9. During the Whitaker test, it is important to remember that a normal renal pelvis pressure is one that is less than _____ cm of water.   9.____

   A. 5   B. 13   C. 22   D. 40

10. The normal pressure in the right atrium is _____ mm Hg. 10.___

   A. 2-8 B. 10-20 C. 20-40 D. 70-100

11. Which of the following embolization materials is NOT pemanently occluding? 11.___

   A. Gelfoam
   C. Detachable balloons
   B. Absolute ethanol
   D. Bucrylate

12. Which of the following radiographic projections would typically be used to view the distal left main coronary artery? 12.___

   A. 10° RAO
   C. 30° LAO
   B. 20°-30° cranial
   D. Left lateral/10° caudal

13. For arteriography of the arm, a #_____ French catheter is MOST appropriate. 13.___

   A. 2 B. 5 C. 8 D. 14

14. Contrast media delivery rate is inversely proportional to the 14.___

   A. catheter caliber
   B. angle of the fixed tip of a catheter
   C. catheter length
   D. number of side holes in a catheter

Questions 15-21.

DIRECTIONS: Questions 15 through 21 refer to the figure shown on the following page, a frontal diagram of the distribution of the superior mesenteric artery. Place the letter that corresponds to each artery in the space at the right.

15. Marginal artery 15.____
16. Left colic artery 16.____
17. Ileocolic artery 17.____
18. Jejunal and ileal arteries 18.____
19. Superior mesenteric artery 19.____
20. Middle colic artery 20.____
21. Right colic artery 21.____

22. The time required for the electronics in an automatic film changer to respond is known as _____ time.

    A. down
    B. flex
    C. phase-in
    D. zero

23. Which of the following radiographic projections is BEST suited for visualizing the inferior mesenteric artery?

    A. Left lateral
    B. 20°-30° RPO
    C. 45° LAO
    D. 15° LPO

24. Each of the following is typically involved in a biliary stone removal procedure EXCEPT

    A. general anesthesia
    B. contrast media
    C. fluoroscopy
    D. catheterization

25. When myocardial ischemia occurs during coronary angio-graphy, the MOST common response is to

    A. perform left ventriculogram before coronary angiography
    B. interrupt pre-catheterization heparin infusion
    C. remove catheter from coronary ostium and suspend injections
    D. reverse heparin at the completion of the procedure

KEY (CORRECT ANSWERS)

1. B
2. D
3. C
4. C
5. D

6. B
7. B
8. C
9. B
10. A

11. A
12. B
13. B
14. C
15. R

16. S
17. V
18. W
19. T
20. Q

21. U
22. D
23. D
24. A
25. C

TEST 3

DIRECTIONS: Each question or incomplete statement is followed by several suggested answers or completions. Select the one that BEST answers the question or completes the statement. *PRINT THE LETTER OF THE CORRECT ANSWER IN THE SPACE AT THE RIGHT.*

1. For performing a nephrostomy, the BEST patient position is 1.____
   A. RAO B. RPO C. supine D. prone

2. A _____ is a percutaneous needle puncture drainage procedure. 2.____
   A. liver biopsy B. splenic arteriogram
   C. lymphangiogram D. nephrostomy

3. For visualizing the symmetry of the pulmonary arteries, the MOST common position is 3.____
   A. RPO B. AP C. PA D. LAO

4. Each of the following is a condition that may predispose a patient to peripheral arterial embolism EXCEPT 4.____
   A. bacterial endocarditis
   B. atrial fibrillation
   C. ventricular depolarization
   D. recurrent cardiac arrhythmias

5. Typically, single-rescuer CPR involves the administration of single breaths at an interval of _____ seconds. 5.____
   A. 2 B. 5 C. 10 D. 30

6. Which of the following is NOT a risk commonly associated with percutaneous transephatic biliary drainage? 6.____
   A. Bleeding
   B. Undesirable biliary migration
   C. Pneumothorax
   D. Sepsis

7. Which of the following steps in forming a digital angiographic image occurs FIRST? 7.____
   A. Image is scanned by electron beam from top to bottom
   B. X-rays converted into 2-diraensional visible light on the output phosphor
   C. Conversion to electronic video signal
   D. Image is focused onto video camera pickup tube

8. What type of guidewire is used for vessel entry prior to iliac angioplasty? 8.____
   A. Straight B. Standard J
   C. Long-tapered D. Bentson

9. A foreign object casts a shadow that is 5.4 cm wide on a PA abdomen radiograph produced at 100 cm. The mass is located 4.4 cm from the film. What is the magnification factor? 9.____
   A. 0.96 B. 1.01 C. 1.05 D. 1.07

10. Existing cardiovascular disease should be a contraindication for a pre-injection dose of
    A. ephedrine
    B. prednisone
    C. epinephrine
    D. nifedipine

11. Which of the following end systolic volumes, in ml/m^2, of the left ventricle falls within the normal adult range?
    A. 25
    B. 46
    C. 64
    D. 89

12. The outer portion of a basic arterial puncture needle is known as the
    A. pith
    B. obturator
    C. torque surface
    D. cannula

13. The Judkins technique is performed for the purpose of
    A. insertion of plastic endoprostheses
    B. cannulation of the left coronary ostium
    C. antegrade pyelography
    D. inferior venocaval filter placement

14. Coronary circulation is left-dominant in about _____% of all patients.
    A. 8
    B. 32
    C. 50
    D. 72

15. What is the approximate injection rate of contrast material, in ml/sec, used for an inferior venocavogram?
    A. 6-10
    B. 12-15
    C. 20
    D. 35

16. _____ is an agent that may be used both before and after an angioplasty procedure.
    A. Vasopressin
    B. Ephedrine
    C. Atropine
    D. Heparin

17. The pulmonary artery rises from the
    A. left atrium
    B. left ventricle
    C. right atrium
    D. right ventricle

18. In ultrasound cardiac imaging, most adult patients are imaged with the use of _____ MHz transducers.
    A. 1
    B. 3.5
    C. 5
    D. 7.5

19. The film sequence *3/sec x 3 sec: 1/sec x 3-5 sec* would MOST likely be used for
    A. celiac arteriography
    B. lower limb venography
    C. ventriculography
    D. pulmonary arteriography

20. Of the 12 standard ECG leads, which of the following is indirect and bipolar?
    A. aV$_R$
    B. V$_3$
    C. III
    D. aV$_F$

21. Cerebral venous drainage is provided by each of the following EXCEPT 21.____

    A. internal jugular vein
    B. dural sinuses
    C. subdural sinuses
    D. cerebral veins

22. If the filming sequence for a splenic angiogram is extended, which of the following structures will be visualized? 22.____

    A. Portal vein
    B. Sigmoid arteries
    C. Superior mesenteric artery
    D. Inferior mesenteric artery

23. Which of the following angiographic applications would typically require the contrast material of LOWEST concentration? 23.____

    A. Selective cerebral vessel
    B. Angiocardiogram
    C. Aortic arch
    D. Subclavian artery

24. For angiography involving the left coronary artery, automatic pressure injectors should typically be preset at _____ ml/sec. 24.____

    A. 2-3   B. 3-4   C. 4-6   D. 5-7

25. For visualizing lesions in the iliac or common femoral arteries, which patient position if probably BEST? 25.____

    A. AP   B. PA   C. Oblique   D. Supine

KEY (CORRECT ANSWERS)

1. D		11. A	
2. D		12. D	
3. B		13. B	
4. C		14. A	
5. B		15. C	
6. B		16. D	
7. B		17. C	
8. B		18. B	
9. C		19. D	
10. A		20. C	

21. C
22. A
23. A
24. B
25. C

TEST 4

DIRECTIONS: Each question or incomplete statement is followed by several suggested answers or completions. Select the one that BEST answers the question or completes the statement. *PRINT THE LETTER OF THE CORRECT ANSWER IN THE SPACE AT THE RIGHT.*

1. Pulmonary hypertension is described as *severe* if pulmonary artery pressure is AT LEAST _____ mm Hg.

    A. 30   B. 50   C. 70   D. 80

2. Which of the following is NOT typically a factor predisposing a patient to arterial thrombosis?

    A. Long duration of catheterization
    B. Movable-care catheters
    C. Improper compression of puncture site
    D. Multiple puncture attempts

3. For the placement of a Vena-Tech filter, the BEST approach is through the

    A. left femoral vein
    B. right femoral vein
    C. left femoral artery
    D. right femoral artery

4. The purpose of a cardiac transducer is to

    A. measure cardiac input
    B. measure ventricular volume
    C. measure ventricular pressure
    D. monitor the ECG system

5. Which of the following procedures will typically require the LOWEST total dosage of intravascular contrast media?

    A. Vertebral cerebral arteriography
    B. Pulmonary arteriography
    C. Thoracic aortography
    D. Hepatic arteriography

6. Severe allergic reactions to contrast agents are BEST prevented by AT LEAST _____ hours of premedication.

    A. 6-12   B. 18-24   C. 24-48   D. 48-72

7. The _____ artery should be used as a puncture site for femoral arteriography if both femoral pulses are absent.

    A. right axillary
    B. left axillary
    C. right brachial
    D. left brachial

8. In order to avoid cyanosis in an adult, the patient should take AT LEAST _____ breaths per minute.

    A. 5   B. 10   C. 15   D. 20

9. Typically, an inferior vena cava filter is placed

   A. inferior to the renal veins
   B. between the renal and hepatic veins
   C. superior to the common iliac bifurcation
   D. superior to the splenic vein

10. Each of the following is a hemodynamic consequence of the injection of contrast media EXCEPT

    A. increased cardiac output
    B. vasodilation
    C. leveling of P wave
    D. increased heart rate

11. Simultaneous cine recording and viewing of a fluoroscopic image can be achieved by using a

    A. beam splitting mirror
    B. grid-biased x-ray tube
    C. digital image display
    D. low-frequency generator

12. What is the term for a drop in overall catheter tip pressure?

    A. Attenuation
    B. Inversion
    C. Damping
    D. Extension

13. Of the following embolization techniques, which will last the SHORTEST amount of time?

    A. Gelfoam
    B. Gianturco coils
    C. Absolute ethanol
    D. Autologous clot

14. The normal peak systolic pressure in the left ventricle is _____ mm Hg.

    A. 5-10   B. 30-50   C. 60-80   D. 100-140

15. A patient complains of having *tongue thickness* after an injection of contrast media. Which of the following should be administered?

    A. Anesthetic
    B. Heparin
    C. Amphetamine
    D. Antihistamine

16. The maximum outer diameter of balloons used for PTC angioplasty is APPROXIMATELY _____ mm.

    A. 3-4   B. 5-7   C. 6-8   D. 8-10

17. If the femoral approach is ill-advised or impossible for thoracic aortography, what approach is favored?

    A. Brachial   B. Axillary   C. Aortic   D. Subclavian

18. Atrial arrhythmias that occur during cardiac catheterization are generally.

    A. heart blocks
    B. sinus rhythms
    C. bradycardias
    D. fibrillations

19. Which of the following filming sequences would MOST likely be used for ventriculography?

    A. 3/sec x 2 sec: l/sec x 2 sec: 2 delays
    B. 2/sec x 5-10 sec
    C. 3/sec x 3 sec: l/sec x 3 sec: 2 delays
    D. Cine

20. Under the conditions of strict isolation, each of the following must be worn EXCEPT

    A. mask   B. gloves   C. hood   D. gown

21. During vasodilation procedures, the approximate MINIMUM peripheral artery pressure should be _____ mm Hg.

    A. 20   B. 60   C. 80   D. 120

22. The QRS complex of an ECG measures

    A. recovery
    B. ventricular depolarization
    C. atrial depolarization
    D. sinus rhythm

23. Prior to an angiographic procedure, coagulation assessment is mandated when visceral transit by anything larger than a _____-gauge needle is anticipated.

    A. 12   B. 16   C. 22   D. 28

24. Each of the following is a specific indication that normally requires the use of a low-osmolar contrast agent EXCEPT

    A. history of prior allergic reaction to ionic contrast
    B. ulcer or gastrointestinal bleeding
    C. internal mammary injection
    D. baseline renal insufficiency

25. For a renal angiogram, which of the following TOTAL doses, in ml, of contrast material would be within the recommended procedural average?

    A. 10   B. 30   C. 100   D. 140

KEY (CORRECT ANSWERS)

1. C
2. B
3. B
4. C
5. A

6. B
7. B
8. B
9. A
10. C

11. A
12. C
13. D
14. D
15. D

16. A
17. B
18. D
19. D
20. C

21. A
22. B
23. C
24. B
25. B

EXAMINATION SECTION
TEST 1

DIRECTIONS: Each question or incomplete statement is followed by several suggested answers or completions. Select the one that BEST answers the question or completes the statement. *PRINT THE LETTER OF THE CORRECT ANSWER IN THE SPACE AT THE RIGHT.*

1. Which one of the following is an indication for cardiac catheterization?

    A. Acute myocardial ischemia
    B. Angina pectoris
    C. Fever/infection
    D. Renal failure

2. In the anteroposterior position, the right atrium of the heart lies _____ and is the _____ border of the heart.

    A. anteriorly; left
    B. anteriorly; right
    C. posteriorly; left
    D. posteriorly; right

3. In coronary arteriography, if the aorta is not dilated or is of average size, most angiographers would start with a Judkins left coronary catheter JL

    A. 3   B. 4   C. 5   D. 6

4. The central nervous system drug that alleviates modest to oppressive pain best describes

    A. antianxiety drugs
    B. antidepressants
    C. narcotics
    D. sedatives

5. In selective coronary arteriography of the left coronary artery, which position is also known as the *spider* view, and provides for visualization of the proximal left anterior descending, the left main coronary artery, and the proximal circumflex artery?

    A. Anteroposterior position
    B. Lateral position
    C. Left anterior oblique position with caudal angulation
    D. Right anterior oblique position with caudal angulation

6. Right ventricular pressure is normally _____ mmHg systolic and less than _____ mmHg end-diastolic.

    A. 7 to 10; 2
    B. 15 to 30; 7
    C. 70 to 100; 20
    D. 150 to 300; 70

7. The peripheral nervous system drug that encourages blood clotting is termed a(n)

    A. anticoagulant
    B. analgesic
    C. hemostatic
    D. vasodilator

8. Which of the following would most likely represent a typical angiographic generator?

    A. 400 to 800 mA; 50 to 80 kVp
    B. 400 to 800 mA; 50 to 100+ kVp

C. 800 to 1500 mA; 50 to 80 kVp
D. 800 to 1500 mA; 50 to 100+ kVp

9. A _____ device is often used for angiography of the arterial structures of the lower extremities, permitting movement of the angiographic table resulting in a sequence of images.

   A. grid   B. roll film   C. stepping   D. wedge

10. Which of the following best defines the number of cubic centimeters of contrast media delivered each second?

    A. Delay rate   B. Flow rate
    C. Pressure rate rise   D. Total volume rate

11. Increased aortic systolic and diastolic pressures might indicate which of the following?
    I. Aortic insufficiency
    II. Patent ductus arteriosus
    III. Poor ventricular outflow
    The CORRECT answer is:

    A. I, II   B. I, III
    C. II, III   D. I, II, III

12. Ventricular septal defects are usually noted as a loud murmur

    A. at birth
    B. 2 weeks to 2 months
    C. 2 months to 2 years
    D. typically not before 2 years of age

13. Which of the following is the BEST reason describing why ionic contrast has a higher incidence of reaction?

    A. Higher osmolarity   B. Lower osmolarity
    C. Less iodine   D. More iodine

14. The *gold standard* for detecting pulmonary emboli is a(n)

    A. chest x-ray
    B. nuclear medicine perfusion scan
    C. pulmonary angiography
    D. ultrasonography

15. Which of the following is the largest single cause of aortic dissection?

    A. Hypertension   B. Hypotension
    C. Marfan's syndrome   D. Pregnancy

16. Who is responsible for securing informed consent?

    A. Chief technologist   B. Nurse
    C. Physician   D. Technologist

17. Which of the following organs would most likely be damaged following rapid administration of contrast media leading to overdose and toxicity?

    I. Brain
    II. Kidneys
    III. Liver

    The CORRECT answer is:

    A. I, II　　　B. I, III　　　C. II, III　　　D. I, II, III

18. The titanium Greenfield vena cava filter is often used to prevent _____ and is also known as a _____ filter.

    A. hemorrhage; balloon
    B. hemorrhage; umbrella
    C. pulmonary emboli from reaching the lungs; balloon
    D. pulmonary emboli from reaching the lungs; umbrella

19. Which one of the following would NOT be considered a bronchodilator?

    A. Acetaminophen　　　B. Albuterol
    C. Ephedrine　　　D. Epinephrine

20. Which one of the following is often called a sucking chest wound?

    A. Closed pneumothorax　　　B. Hemopneumothorax
    C. Hemothorax　　　D. Open pneumothora

21. What is the average length of time a endotracheal tube or nasal airway can be used?

    A. 1 day　　　B. 5 days　　　C. 3-4 weeks　　　D. No time limit

22. In hypoxia, $PaCO_2$ levels _____, PaO_2 levels _____, and pH _____.

    A. fall; fall; fall　　　B. fall; rise; rise
    C. rise; rise; fall　　　D. rise; fall; fall

23. A patient has periodic loss of consciousness followed by lucid periods. This may represent

    A. epidural hematoma
    B. increased intracranial pressure
    C. spinal cord injury
    D. subdural hematoma

24. Orthostatic (orthoscopic) hypotension, arrhythmia, vascular stenosis, and shock may all lead to

    A. fainting　　　B. focal seizure
    C. grand mal seizure　　　D. petit mal seizure

25. The most common indication of an aortic aneurysm on the plain film PA radiograph is

    A. depression of the diaphragm
    B. elevation of the diaphragm
    C. gross cardiomegaly
    D. mediastinal widening

KEY (CORRECT ANSWERS)

1. B
2. B
3. B
4. C
5. C

6. B
7. C
8. D
9. C
10. B

11. A
12. B
13. A
14. B
15. A

16. C
17. C
18. D
19. A
20. D

21. B
22. D
23. A
24. A
25. C

TEST 2

DIRECTIONS: Each question or incomplete statement is followed by several suggested answers or completions. Select the one that BEST answers the question or completes the statement. *PRINT THE LETTER OF THE CORRECT ANSWER IN THE SPACE AT THE RIGHT.*

1. The normal duration of a surgical scrub would be _____ minutes.
   A. 1 to 2   B. 2 to 3   C. 5 to 10   D. 15 to 30

2. The outer diameter of a No. 6 French catheter would be mm.
   A. 0.2   B. 0.3   C. 2.0   D. 3.0

3. Sterilization and _____ are considered to be synonymous.
   A. antisepsis
   B. bacteriocide
   C. medical asepsis
   D. surgical asepsis

4. In left coronary artery angiography, the circumflex artery would be best shown with a _____ projection.
   A. PA or RAO 5 to 15 degrees
   B. LAO 30 to 40 degrees; cranial 20 to 40 degrees
   C. RAO 20 to 40 degrees
   D. RAO 20 to 40 degrees; caudal 15 to 30 degrees

5. A cardiac gating device will synchronize the injection of contrast medium with the _____ wave impulse of the patient's cardiac cycle.
   A. C   B. Q   C. R   D. S

6. Which of the following types of shock is also known as cold shock, resulting from either a loss of blood volume or plasma volume?
   A. Anaphylactic
   B. Cardiogenic
   C. Hypovolemic
   D. Vasogenic

7. An angiographic suite should be at LEAST _____ times the size of a standard radiographic room.
   A. 2   B. 4   C. 8   D. 16

8. Sterilization and mechanical disinfection will
   A. fail to remove microorganisms and spores
   B. fail to remove both microorganisms and spores
   C. remove both microorganisms and spores
   D. remove microorganisms but not spores

9. If the myocardium contracts normally, but at an elevated rate, this is called
   A. bradycardia
   B. hypercardia
   C. hypocardia
   D. tachycardia

10. Which of the following would most likely be an indication for right ventriculography?

    A. Cardiomyopathy
    B. Mitral valve incompetence
    C. Valvular incompetence
    D. Ventricular septal defects

11. Which method of automatic brightness stabilization in fluoroscopy makes it the most difficult for the operator to choose the method of operation best suited for particular examinations?
    Variable

    A. mA, present kVp
    B. mA with kVp following
    C. kVp with selected mA
    D. kVp, variable mA

12. Which of the following would be a common range of pressure values for an automatic contrast injection device?
    _____ psi.

    A. 5 to 20
    B. 20 to 200
    C. 100 to 1000
    D. 700 to 3000

13. The blurring of the television image (also called stickiness) in fluoroscopic images is called

    A. brightness
    B. contrast
    C. lag
    D. resolution

14. About how much will added filtration decrease skin exposure in fluoroscopy?

    A. 10%   B. 25%   C. 45%   D. 65%

15. Your fluoroscopic boost system raises mA from 2 to 40 mA. Patient exposure will be increased by _____ times.

    A. 2   B. 4   C. 20   D. 40

16. The Inter-Society Commission for Heart Disease Resources recommends a minimum exposure of _____ microroentgens per frame.

    A. 10   B. 20   C. 100   D. 200

17. The most commonly used video disc frame rate is _____ frames/second.

    A. 1   B. 5   C. 15   D. 30

18. Adequate visualization of left ventricular wall motion can be achieved with contrast volumes as small as _____ ml.

    A. 2   B. 20   C. 200   D. 2,000

19. What number is assigned to a no response for any category on the Glasgow Coma Scale?

    A. 1   B. 2   C. 4   D. 5

20. In coronary arteriography, angiographers who use the brachial approach would be most likely to prefer the _____ catheter.

    A. Amplatz   B. Gianturco   C. Judkins   D. Sones

21. The aorta runs a tortuous course in a _____ year-old.

    A. 3   B. 16   C. 45   D. 85

22. In abdominal aortography, the proper delineation of aneurysms and trauma requires the performance of the _____ projections.

    A. AP and lateral
    B. AP and RPO
    C. AP and LPO
    D. RPO and LPO

23. Which of the following statements is NOT true regarding mesenteric angiography?

    A. In an acute GI bleed, the suspected vessel is injected first.
    B. If lower GI hemorrhage is suspected, the pelvic region should be investigated first.
    C. Filming should be rapid during the arterial flow.
    D. Digital subtraction angiography is preferred for ill or uncooperative patients.

24. Expected kVp and exposure time for visceral angiography of the adult would be _____ kVp and _____ ms.

    A. 70; 10   B. 70; 100   C. 100; 10   D. 100; 100

25. In visceral angiography, the patient may have to hold his/her breath for _____ seconds.

    A. 2-3   B. 3-5   C. 25-35   D. 45-75

KEY (CORRECT ANSWERS)

1. C
2. C
3. D
4. D
5. C
6. C
7. A
8. D
9. D
10. C
11. D
12. C
13. C
14. D
15. C
16. B
17. D
18. A
19. A
20. D
21. D
22. A
23. D
24. B
25. C

TEST 3

DIRECTIONS: Each question or incomplete statement is followed by several suggested answers or completions. Select the one that BEST answers the question or completes the statement. *PRINT THE LETTER OF THE CORRECT ANSWER IN THE SPACE AT THE RIGHT.*

1. Which of the following is most likely an indication for hepatic angiography? 1.___

    A. Atherosclerotic disease   B. Budd-Chiari syndrome
    C. Therapeutic embolization   D. Wilms' tumor

2. Which visceral organ differs from the others in that it has a dual blood supply? 2.___

    A. Kidney   B. Liver   C. Pancreas   D. Spleen

3. Which one of the following is NOT drained by the portal venous system? 3.___

    A. Colon   B. Kidneys   C. Pancreas   D. Spleen

4. Which abdominal organ is most frequently damaged in automobile accidents? 4.___

    A. Colon   B. Kidneys   C. Spleen   D. Stomach

5. Which of the following is the LEAST likely reason for performing a renal arteriogram? 5.___

    A. Delineation of a cyst
    B. Diagnosis of renal tumors
    C. Evaluation of renovascular hypertension
    D. Preoperative assessment of donor kidneys for renal transplant

6. Most commonly, adults will exhibit how many renal arteries serving each kidney? 6.___

    A. One   B. Two   C. Three   D. Four

7. Of the _____ branches of the celiac trunk, the _____ is the smallest. 7.___

    A. two; left gastric   B. two; splenic
    C. three; left gastric   D. three; splenic

8. Arterial puncture primarily uses the _____ technique. 8.___

    A. common femoral   B. flush
    C. Seldinger   D. selective

9. A deflecting guidewire 9.___

    A. helps by slowing approach
    B. helps by bending straight catheters
    C. is thrombogenic
    D. is not used in visceral angiography

10. In peripheral angiography, if femoral blood flow is incompetent, then a _____ approach is commonly used. 10.___

    A. axillary   B. brachial   C. iliac   D. translumbar

11. Which of the following is NOT true?
    A. Hemorrhage is a definite problem with the translumbar approach.
    B. Selective catheterization of target vessels is difficult with a translumbar approach.
    C. The complication rate of the axillary approach is twice that of the femoral.
    D. The two most frequent techniques used for axillary approach are the angiocath and butterfly.

12. The _____ the catheter used in peripheral angiography, the _____ the potential for thrombus production.
    A. narrower; greater
    B. wider; greater
    C. longer; greater
    D. shorter; greater

13. For a very large patient in aortography, the best solution to a tube overload would be
    A. decreased time
    B. increased time
    C. decreased SID
    D. increased SID

14. In pelvic angiography, the right posterior oblique (RPO) position will best show the _____ internal iliac artery.
    A. left deep femoral artery and the left
    B. left deep femoral artery and the origin of the right
    C. the origin of the right internal iliac artery and the left
    D. right deep femoral artery and the left

15. Which of the following is an arterial vasodilator?
    A. Lidocaine
    B. Papaverine
    C. Reserpine
    D. Tolazoline (priscoline)

16. Which of the following is most likely the minimum program run for a patient having lower extremity angiography and a rapid flow rate? _____ seconds.
    A. 5
    B. 25
    C. 50
    D. 65

17. The most common guidewire configuration is the
    A. C
    B. I
    C. J
    D. L

18. Thrombogenecity of guidewires is reduced with the use of
    A. heparin
    B. lidocaine
    C. stainless steel
    D. Teflon

19. Guidewires used on adults are typically _____ mm in length.
    A. 45
    B. 100
    C. 145
    D. 200

20. For translumbar aortography, the patient is usually placed in the _____ position.
    A. LPO
    B. lateral
    C. prone
    D. RPO

21. Complete demonstration of the blood vessels from the pelvis to the foot when using a stepping table usually takes

    A. 5 to 10 seconds
    B. 25 to 35 seconds
    C. 1 to 2 minutes
    D. 2 to 4 minutes

22. Which of the following would probably be the MINIMUM speed film-screen combination for aortography and extremity runoff?

    A. 100
    B. 200
    C. 400
    D. 800

23. The most constant control of contrast media administration for venography would be a _____ injection.

    A. drip
    B. hand
    C. rapid power
    D. slow power

24. Which one of the following is NOT an indication for cerebral angiography?

    A. Aneurysm
    B. Cerebral hemorrhage
    C. Presurgical evaluation
    D. Severe hypertension

25. Which one of the following is NOT an anterior branch of the external carotid artery?

    A. Facial
    B. Internal maxillary
    C. Pharyngeal
    D. Superior thyroid

KEY (CORRECT ANSWERS)

1.	B	11.	D
2.	B	12.	A
3.	B	13.	C
4.	C	14.	B
5.	A	15.	D
6.	A	16.	B
7.	C	17.	C
8.	C	18.	A
9.	B	19.	C
10.	A	20.	C

21. B
22. D
23. B
24. D
25. C

TEST 4

DIRECTIONS: Each question or incomplete statement is followed by several suggested answers or completions. Select the one that BEST answers the question or completes the statement. *PRINT THE LETTER OF THE CORRECT ANSWER IN THE SPACE AT THE RIGHT.*

1. Which one of the following would NOT be considered to be part of the cervical portion of the internal carotid artery?
   Carotid

   A. bifurcation   B. body   C. siphon   D. sinus

   1._____

2. For the purpose of serial magnification in cerebral angio-graphy, a _____ mm focal spot should be used.

   A. 0.3   B. 0.6   C. 0.9   D. 1.2

   2._____

3. The right and left pontine are branches of the _____ artery.

   A. basilar   B. left subclavian
   C. left vertebral   D. right subclavian

   3._____

4. For biplane serial filming in cerebral angiography, a _____ grid is used for the horizontal film and a _____ for the vertical film.

   A. 4:1 linear; 4:1 crossed   B. 4:1 crossed; 4:1 linear
   C. 8:1 linear; 8:1 crossed   D. 8:1 crossed; 8:1 linear

   4._____

5. What film screen speed combination is typically used for cerebral angiography?

   A. 100 to 250   B. 300 to 550
   C. 600 to 850   D. 900 to 1200

   5._____

6. What two things will citrates in a contrast medium do?
   Increase

   A. calcium binding and not be well tolerated by the brain
   B. calcium binding and increase chances of arrhythmias
   C. peripheral discomfort and not be well tolerated by the brain
   D. peripheral discomfort and increase chances of arrhythmias

   6._____

7. In which of the following conditions might the patient experience an *event* in which a *curtain* or *shade* seems to cover one or both eyes for a moment?

   A. Aneurysm
   B. Arteriovenous malformation
   C. Reversible ischemic neurologic defect
   D. Transient ischemic attack

   7._____

8. A *four vessel* study looks at
   I. carotids
   II. subclavians
   III. vertebrals

   The CORRECT answer is:

   A. I, II   B. I, III   C. II, III   D. I, II, III

   8._____

9. The carotid artery would have to be stenosed by _____ % for the stenosis to be considered *hemodynamically significant,* requiring surgery?

    A. 25   B. 50   C. 75   D. 100

10. If the lateral projection on a cerebral angiogram is to demonstrate posterior cerebral circulation, the central should be directed to enter

    A. anterior to the external auditory meatus
    B. anterior and inferior to the external auditory meatus
    C. anterior and superior to the external auditory meatus
    D. behind the external auditory meatus at the mastoid process

11. Which media might be used in the treatment of AVMs and hypervascular renal tumors, that is readily available, inexpensive, and nonviscous?

    A. Absolute ethanol
    B. Hot contrast media
    C. Isobutyl-2-cyanoacrylate
    D. Sodium morrhuate

12. Which one of the following is NOT a contraindication for thrombolysis?

    A. Active internal bleeding
    B. Cerebral artery atherosclerosis
    C. Coagulopathy
    D. Diabetic hemorrhagic retinopathy

13. Which of the following are true regarding streptokinase?
    I. High fibrinolytic ratio
    II. Human derived
    III. Stable at room temperature
    The CORRECT answer is:

    A. I, II   B. I, III
    C. II, III   D. I, II, III

14. Hemangiomas are rarely biopsed due to

    A. high risk of death
    B. lack of cost effectiveness of the procedure
    C. large amount of pain to the patient
    D. low diagnostic ratio of the procedure

15. Which of the following would be classified as ionic contrast media?

    A. Diatrizoate meglumine   B. Iopamidol
    C. Iohexol   D. Metrizamide

16. Which of the following are potential cardiovascular effects of contrast media?
    I. Depressed ST wave segment
    II. Inverted T wave
    III. Lowered T wave
    The CORRECT answer is:

    A. I, II
    B. I, III
    C. II, III
    D. I, II, III

17. During cardiac catheterization, for which of the following changes might the patient be given sublingual nitroglycerin or nifedipine?

    A. Bradycardia/hypotension
    B. Contrast medium reaction
    C. Premature ventricular contraction
    D. ST segment changes

18. Which angiographic procedure has the highest documented death rate?

    A. Abdominal angiography
    B. Cerebral angiography
    C. Pulmonary angiography
    D. Thoracic aortography

19. Most aortic aneurysms occur in the

    A. aortic arch
    B. ascending aorta
    C. descending aorta
    D. thoracic aorta

20. In cerebral angiography, the catheters typically used have

    A. single end hole
    B. single end hole with bilateral side holes
    C. single end hole with multiple side holes
    D. varying assortment of side holes only

21. Which of the following is most likely a normal hemoglobin level? _____ g/dl.

    A. 7
    B. 14
    C. 28
    D. 56

22. The tip of the catheter is placed at the level of _____ for abdominal aortography.

    A. T-8
    B. T-10
    C. T-12
    D. L-2

23. Visualization of the upper extremity from subclavian to digital arteries will usually involve

    A. a single injection
    B. increased amounts of contrast media
    C. larger film sizes
    D. multiple injections

24. For antiplatelet therapy for balloon angioplasty, the patient might be prescribed _____ mg of aspirin four times a day.

    A. 300
    B. 600
    C. 1200
    D. 2400

25. Which of the following are percutaneous approaches commonly used to place an inferior vena cava filter?   25.____
    I. Axillary
    II. Femoral
    III. Right jugular
    The CORRECT answer is:

    A. I, II
    C. II, III
    B. I, III
    D. I, II, III

KEY (CORRECT ANSWERS)

1. C
2. A
3. A
4. C
5. C

6. B
7. C
8. B
9. C
10. D

11. A
12. B
13. B
14. C
15. A

16. D
17. D
18. D
19. B
20. A

21. B
22. C
23. D
24. A
25. D

TEST 5

DIRECTIONS: Each question or incomplete statement is followed by several suggested answers or completions. Select the one that BEST answers the question or completes the statement. *PRINT THE LETTER OF THE CORRECT ANSWER IN THE SPACE AT THE RIGHT.*

1. Place the steps of the Seldinger technique in the correct order.
    I. Insertion of guide wire
    II. Insertion of needle
    III. Removal of guide wire
    IV. Removal of needle
    V. Placement of needle in lumen of vessel
    VI. Threading of catheter to area of interest
   The CORRECT answer is:

   A. I, II, III, IV, V, VI
   B. II, I, III, IV, V, VI
   C. II, V, I, IV, VI, III
   D. IV, V, VI, I, III, II

   1.____

2. To achieve 2x magnification during a cerebral angiogram for the lateral projection, using a 100 cm (40 inch) SID, place the patient's head _____ the film.

   A. directly against
   B. 10 inches from
   C. 20 inches from
   D. 30 inches from

   2.____

3. What is the range of high-concentration contrast medium typically used for thoracic aortography?
   _____ cc.

   A. 10 to 20   B. 20 to 40   C. 40 to 80   D. 80 to 160

   3.____

4. Which position for thoracic aortography tends to be most useful in demonstrating the arch or great vessel branch deformities?

   A. AP   B. Lateral   C. LPO   D. RPO

   4.____

5. Which of the following best describes the typical delivery rate for contrast for selective renal angiography?
   _____ cc at a rate of _____ cc per second.

   A. 6 to 10; 5 to 6
   B. 15 to 25; 8 to 12
   C. 35 to 45; 14 to 16
   D. 45 to 65; 25

   5.____

6. A filming rate of 2 films/second for 4 seconds, followed by 1 film/second for 2 seconds, and 1 film every other
   1 second for 8 seconds best describes

   A. abdominal angiography
   B. lower limb arteriography
   C. renal angiography
   D. splenoportography

   6.____

7. Which of the following is the most common contraindication for peripheral angiography?

   A. Adverse reaction to contrast media
   B. Local infection

   7.____

95

C. Phlebitis
D. Thrombosis

8. If a lower limb arteriogram requires abdominal radiographs, _____ cc of high concentration contrast is used at a rate of _____ cc/second.

   A. 10-20; 8-10
   B. 10-20; 10-15
   C. 40-60; 8-10
   D. 40-60; 10-15

9. Which of the following is NOT a method used to increase the rate of blood flow for patients with poor circulation undergoing lower limb arteriography?

   A. Administration of a double dose of contrast
   B. Blood pressure cuff
   C. Exercise
   D. Tolazoline

10. Injecting 15 cc of a 45 to 60% concentration of contrast medium at a rate of 7 to 8 cc/second best describes which of the following procedures?

    A. Abdominal angiography
    B. Lower limb arteriography
    C. Lower limb venography
    D. Splenoportography

11. Which of the following is best described as a cage-like metal device placed in a vessel to enlarge the lumen?

    A. Infusion catheter
    B. Pulse spray catheter
    C. Retrieval basket
    D. Stent

12. What is the expected life expectancy (in terms of vessel patency) for balloon catheter vessel dilation?

    A. 1-2 years
    B. 3-5 years
    C. 7-10 years
    D. Indeterminable

13. Frontal positioning for the vertebrobasilar angiogram involves maintaining a _____ angle between the central ray and the EAM, with the central ray passing through the level of the EAM.

    A. 10 degrees caudal
    B. 30 degrees caudal
    C. 10 degrees cephalad
    D. 30 degrees cephalad

14. The subclavian continues to become the _____ artery, which gives rise to the _____ artery.

    A. axillary; brachial
    B. brachial; axillary
    C. radial; ulnar
    D. ulnar; radial

15. This originates from the aorta at about the 3rd lumbar vertebra, 3 or 4 cm above the level of the bifurcation of the common iliac arteries.

    A. Inferior mesenteric artery
    B. Left renal artery
    C. Right renal artery
    D. Superior mesenteric artery

16. The internal carotid artery supplies primarily the _____ portion of the brain.

    A. anterior   B. inferior   C. posterior   D. superior

17. In thoracic aortography, the LPO position will best show
    I. arch
    II. coarctation
    III. patent ductus arteriosus
    The CORRECT answer is:

    A. I, II   B. I, III
    C. II, III   D. I, II, III

18. A 3 ml/sec injection for a 15 ml total volume of contrast media best describes _____ arteriogram.

    A. celiac   B. inferior mesenteric
    C. splenic   D. superior mesenteric

19. In central venography, collimation to the long axis of the vena cava _____ image quality _____ visualization of peripheral or collateral veins.

    A. improves; and improves
    B. improves; but may prevent
    C. decreases; but improves
    D. decreases; and may prevent

20. Which of the following are types of vascular access devices?
    I. Implanted
    II. Nontunneled
    III. Tunneled
    The CORRECT answer is:

    A. I, II   B. I, III
    C. II, III   D. I, II, III

21. Which one of the following is NOT true regarding cerebral circulation time?

    A. Arterial spasms can shorten transit time.
    B. Arteriovenous malformations shorten transit time.
    C. Circulation time is slightly prolonged by the use of contrast media.
    D. Intracranial pressure may cause a delay in transit time.

22. Which of the following would be considered a permanent embolization agent?

    A. Gelfoam
    B. Gianturco stainless steel coils
    C. Microfibrillar collagen
    D. Vasoconstrictors

23. If the aortic arch is normal but the descending aorta extends downward and to the right, this is known as

    A. inverse aorta   B. left circumflex aorta
    C. pseudocoarctation   D. right circumflex aorta

24. The inferior mesenteric vein does NOT open into the splenic vein, instead ending at the angle of union of the splenic and superior mesenteric arteries, in about _____% of cases.   24.____

    A. 10   B. 20   C. 40   D. 80

25. The air gap significantly reduces scatter reaching the film by   25.____

    A. *decreasing* the source-image receptor distance (SID)
    B. *increasing* the SID
    C. *decreasing* the object-image receptor distance (OID)
    D. *increasing* the OID

KEY (CORRECT ANSWERS)

1. C
2. C
3. C
4. D
5. A

6. A
7. A
8. D
9. A
10. B

11. D
12. B
13. B
14. A
15. A

16. A
17. C
18. B
19. B
20. D

21. A
22. B
23. B
24. A
25. D

CARDIOVASCULAR SYSTEMS
EXAMINATION SECTION
TEST 1

DIRECTIONS: Each question or incomplete statement is followed by several suggested answers or completions. Select the one that BEST answers the question or completes the statement. *PRINT THE LETTER OF THE CORRECT ANSWER IN THE SPACE AT THE RIGHT.*

1. The wall of the heart is made up of all of the following EXCEPT the   1.____

   A. pericardium
   C. myocardium
   B. epicardium
   D. endocardium

2. Among the following statements, the one which is TRUE regarding the pericardium is: 2.____

   A. It contains about 30 ml of serous fluid
   B. It is tough and fibrous and does not readily stretch
   C. If more than 100 ml of fluid accumulates within the pericardium, it may compromise heart contractility
   D. All of the above

3. The MAIN function of the heart is to   3.____

   A. transport the waste products of metabolism to the cells
   B. deliver oxygenated blood and nutrients to every cell in the body
   C. deliver non-oxygenated blood to the cells in the body
   D. deliver chemical messages to the cells

4. Of the following, the structure which collects non-oxygenated blood returning from the body is the   4.____

   A. left atrium
   C. right atrium
   B. right ventricle
   D. left ventricle

5. The vessels that carry blood to the heart are   5.____

   A. arteries
   C. capillaries
   B. arterioles
   D. veins

6. It is NOT true that the heart   6.____

   A. weighs about 300 grams in males and 250 grams in females
   B. is usually 10-12 cm long
   C. is usually located in the right mediastinum
   D. is usually 9 cm wide and 6 cm thick

7. The MOST common location of atria is in the _____ portion of the heart.   7.____

   A. superior
   C. middle
   B. inferior
   D. all of the above

8. The MOST common location and function of the superior vena cava are that it is located _____ and drains _____.

   A. at the right side of the heart; unoxygenated blood from the upper body
   B. at the left side of the heart; oxygenated blood from the lower body
   C. on the right side; unoxygenated blood from the lower part of the body
   D. in the right atrium; blood from the heart itself

9. The high-pressure pump that drives blood OUT of the heart against the relatively high resistance of the systemic arteries is called the

   A. right atrium
   B. left atrium
   C. left ventricle
   D. right ventricle

10. Oxygenated blood is usually supplied to the heart via the _____ artery (arteries).

    A. carotid
    B. coronary
    C. pulmonary
    D. subclavian

11. The MOST accurate definition of cardiac output is:

    A. The amount of blood pumped out by either ventricle, measured in liters per minute
    B. The amount of blood pumped out by either ventricle in a single contraction
    C. The number of cardiac contractions per minute
    D. None of the above

12. The MOST frequent location of the sino atrial node is the _____ near the _____.

    A. right atrium; inlet of the inferior vena cava
    B. right atrium; inlet of the superior vena cava
    C. left atrium; inlet of the pulmonary vein
    D. left ventricle; aortic valve

13. The sinoatrial (SA) node is the fastest pacemaker in the heart, normally firing at the rate of _____ to _____ times per minute.

    A. 20; 40
    B. 40; 60
    C. 60; 100
    D. 100; 300

14. _____ is the process by which muscle fibers are stimulated to contract.

    A. Depolarization
    B. Repolarization
    C. Dyastole
    D. Refractory period

15. The electrolyte that flows into the cell to initiate depolarization is

    A. magnesium
    B. potassium
    C. sodium
    D. phosphate

16. Of the following electrolytes, the one which flows out of the cell to initiate repolarization is

    A. sodium
    B. potassium
    C. calcium
    D. magnesium

17. Depolarization of the atria produces which of the following waves on the ECG? A(n)

    A. P wave
    B. T wave
    C. QRS complex
    D. N wave

18. Of the following waves, repolarization of the atria and ventricles produces _____ on the ECG.   18.____

    A. QRS complex   B. P waves
    C. T waves   D. none of the above

19. The coronary arteries   19.____

    A. originate from the base of the ascending aorta
    B. are above the leaflets of the aortic valve
    C. provide blood supply to the cardiac muscles
    D. all of the above

20. All of the following are caused by the stimulation of beta receptors EXCEPT   20.____

    A. bronchoconstriction
    B. increased heart rate
    C. increased heart contractability
    D. vasodilation

21. Alpha receptor stimulation does NOT cause   21.____

    A. vasoconstriction   B. bronchoconstriction
    C. no effect on the heart   D. increased heart rate

22. Which of the following is pure beta agonist?   22.____

    A. Isoproterenol   B. Metaraminol
    C. Norepinephrine   D. Dopamine

23. The agent of choice to treat increased blood pressure when hypotension has been caused by neurogenic shock (vasodilation) is   23.____

    A. isoproterenol   B. atropin
    C. norepinephrine   D. propranolol

24. Of the following sympathetic agents, the one usually indicated for asystole and anaphylactic shock is   24.____

    A. dopamine   B. epinephrine
    C. metaraminol   D. isoproterenol

25. When used in low doses, this sympathetic agent increases the force of cardiac contraction and helps to maintain urine flow and good perfusion to abdominal organs. This is a description of   25.____

    A. dopamine   B. norepinephrine
    C. metaraminol   D. isoproterenol

4 (#1)

KEY (CORRECT ANSWERS)

1. A
2. D
3. B
4. C
5. D

6. C
7. A
8. A
9. C
10. B

11. A
12. B
13. C
14. A
15. C

16. B
17. A
18. C
19. D
20. A

21. D
22. A
23. C
24. B
25. A

TEST 2

DIRECTIONS: Each question or incomplete statement is followed by several suggested answers or completions. Select the one that BEST answers the question or completes the statement. *PRINT THE LETTER OF THE CORRECT ANSWER IN THE SPACE AT THE RIGHT.*

1. Propranolol is used clinically to

   A. slow the heart rate in certain tachyarrythmias
   B. decrease the pain of chronic angina
   C. decrease irritability in the heart
   D. all of the above

   1.____

2. All of the following are functions of the parasympathetic nervous system EXCEPT

   A. increasing salivation
   B. constricting pupils
   C. slowing the gut
   D. slowing the heart

   2.____

3. Which of the following is NOT a function of the sympathetic nervous system?

   A. Dilate pupils
   B. Increase gut motility
   C. Speed the heart
   D. Constrict blood vessels

   3.____

4. Chest pain is often the presenting sign of acute myocardial infarction. When treating a patient with chest pain, the MOST important question for you to ask him is:

   A. What provoked the pain?
   B. What is the quality and severity of the pain?
   C. Does the pain radiate?
   D. All of the above

   4.____

5. Paroxymal nocturnal dyspnea is one of the classic signs of

   A. pericarditis
   B. right heart failure
   C. left heart failure
   D. asthmatic bronchitis

   5.____

6. The MOST prevalent preventable cause of death in the United States is

   A. diabetes
   B. hypertension
   C. cigarette smoking
   D. high serum cholesterol

   6.____

7. Common sources of risk to the coronary artery include

   A. birth control pills
   B. lack of exercise
   C. male sex
   D. all of the above

   7.____

8. Among the MOST common symptoms of angina pectoris are included

   A. sensations of tightness or pressure
   B. pain induced by anything that increases oxygen requirements
   C. pain radiating to the lower jaw, upper neck, and left shoulder
   D. all of the above

   8.____

9. The difference(s) between the pain of angina pectoris and the pain from acute myocardial infarction is (are) that the pain of acute myocardial infarction

   A. may occur at rest
   B. may last for hours
   C. is not relieved by rest
   D. all of the above

10. All of the following are characteristic of angina pectoris EXCEPT that the pain usually

   A. occurs after exercise, stress and/or cold weather
   B. is relieved by rest
   C. is unresponsive to nitroglycerine
   D. lasts 3 to 5 minutes

11. Among the following, the classic symptoms of acute myocardial infarction include

   A. squeezing or crushing chest pain which is not relieved by rest
   B. a feeling of impending death
   C. diaphoresis, dyspnea, and dizziness
   D. all of the above

12. An elderly patient suffers a sudden onset of dyspnea, hypotension, and confusion. The MOST likely diagnosis is

   A. acute myocardial infarction
   B. angina pectoris
   C. pericarditis
   D. congestive heart failure

13. What is the treatment of choice for angina pectoris?

   A. Propranolol   B. Nitroglycerin
   C. Epinephrine   D. Metaraminol

14. The MAIN goal of treatment for acute myocardial infarction is to

   A. alleviate the patient's fear and pain
   B. prevent the development of serious cardiac dysrhythmias
   C. limit the size of the infarct
   D. all of the above

15. Cardiac work is minimal in the _____ position.

   A. standing   B. sitting
   C. semi-recumbent   D. none of the above

16. _____ therapy is the mainstay of emergency cardiac care.

   A. Epinephrine   B. Oxygen
   C. Propranolol   D. Norepinephrine

17. The proper treatment of uncomplicated acute myocardial infarction en route to the hospital should include all of the following EXCEPT

    A. administering oxygen by mask or nasal cannula
    B. D5W using a 250 ml bag and the infusion rate should be just enough to keep the vein open
    C. giving normal saline bolus
    D. taking blood pressure and repeating at least every 5 minutes

18. In which of the following conditions should the patient be transported before he is stabilized?
    Cardiac

    A. arrest due to uncontrollable hemorrhaging
    B. arrest secondary to cold exposure
    C. rhythms that require immediate pacemaker insertion
    D. all of the above

19. The preferred pain medication for treating a hypotensive patient with acute myocardial infarction is

    A. morphine sulphate
    B. nitrous oxide
    C. codeine
    D. acetominophen

20. Of the following medications, the one you should draw BEFORE administering morphine to a patient with an acute myocardial infarction is

    A. atropine sulphate
    B. nitroglycerine
    C. propranolol
    D. digoxin

21. It would be acceptable to administer morphine to a patient suffering from

    A. low blood pressure
    B. bronchial asthma
    C. AMI involving the inferior wall of the heart
    D. hypertension and pulmonary edema

22. Criteria for thrombolytic therapy for acute myocardial infarction includes all of the following EXCEPT

    A. recent CPR
    B. alert patient who is able to give informed consent
    C. age between 30 and 75 years
    D. chest pain lasting more than 20 minutes but less than 6 hours

23. Common signs and symptoms of left heart failure include

    A. extreme restlessness and agitation
    B. severe dyspnea and tachypnea
    C. frothy pink sputum
    D. all of the above

24. Which of the following heart chambers is MOST commonly damaged by acute myocardial infarction?

    A. Right ventricle
    B. Left ventricle
    C. Left atrium
    D. Right atrium

25. Of the following medications, the one(s) which should be drawn up ready, pending the physician's order for administration, for the treatment of left heart failure is (are)

    A. morphine sulphate
    B. furosemide
    C. digoxin
    D. all of the above

Questions 26-30.

DIRECTIONS: In Questions 26 through 30, match the numbered description with the lettered part of the circulatory system, as listed in Column I, to which it is most closely related. Place the letter of the CORRECT answer in the appropriate space at the right.

COLUMN I
A. Epicardium
B. Endocardium
C. Myocardium
D. Pericardium
E. Coronary sinus

26. The tough fibrous sac which surrounds the heart.

27. The outermost layer of the heart wall.

28. The innermost layer of the heart wall.

29. The middle layer of the heart wall.

30. A large vessel in the posterior part of the coronary sulcus into which venous blood empties.

KEY (CORRECT ANSWERS)

1.	D	16.	B
2.	C	17.	C
3.	B	18.	D
4.	D	19.	B
5.	C	20.	A
6.	C	21.	D
7.	D	22.	A
8.	D	23.	D
9.	D	24.	B
10.	C	25.	D
11.	D	26.	D
12.	A	27.	A
13.	B	28.	B
14.	D	29.	C
15.	C	30.	E

TEST 3

DIRECTIONS: Each question or incomplete statement is followed by several suggested answers or completions. Select the one that BEST answers the question or completes the statement. *PRINT THE LETTER OF THE CORRECT ANSWER IN THE SPACE AT THE RIGHT.*

1. Pre-hospital treatment of left heart failure would NOT include 1.___

    A. administration of beta blocker
    B. administration of 100% oxygen
    C. seating the patient with his feet dangling
    D. starting an intravenous line with D5W

2. The MOST common cause of right heart failure is 2.___

    A. cor pulmonale
    B. tricuspid stenosis
    C. left heart failure
    D. cardiac tamponade

3. All of the following can occur as a result of ventricle failure EXCEPT 3.___

    A. blood backs up into the vein
    B. back-up increases the venous pressure
    C. back-up decreases the venous pressure
    D. blood serum escapes into the tissue and produces edema

4. Signs and symptoms of right heart failure do NOT include 4.___

    A. collapsed jugular vein
    B. hepatosplenomegaly
    C. peripheral edema
    D. tachycardia

5. Common signs and symptoms of cardiogenic shock include all of the following EXCEPT 5.___

    A. pulse racing and thready
    B. severe hypertension
    C. respiration rapid and shallow
    D. confused or comatose state

6. The differentiating factor(s) between the pain of a dissecting aneurysm and an acute myocardial infarction is (are) that the pain of a dissecting aneurysm 6.___

    A. is maximal from the outset
    B. is often included in the back between the shoulder blades
    C. does not abate once it has started
    D. all of the above

7. A 60-year-old male has sudden back pain and a pulsatile abdominal mass. Ten minutes later, his blood pressure starts dropping. 7.___
Pre-hospital management for this patient would include all of the following EXCEPT

    A. administering oxygen
    B. stabilizing the patient before transport
    C. applying (but not inflating) the mast
    D. starting an IV en route with normal saline or lactated ringer's

8. A 35-year-old comatose male has cold and clammy skin, shallow breathing, and thready pulse.
   The FIRST thing you should do to treat this patient is

   A. start an IV D5W
   B. apply monitoring electrodes
   C. secure an open airway
   D. administer epinephrine

9. The MOST common complications of hypertension include

   A. renal damage
   B. stroke
   C. heart failure
   D. all of the above

10. Acute hypertensive crisis is usually signaled by a sudden marked rise in blood pressure to a level greater than _____ mmHg.

    A. 120/80
    B. 140/80
    C. 200/130
    D. none of the above

11. Which of the following is the drug of choice for treatment of hypertensive encephalopathy?

    A. Propranolol
    B. Diazoxide
    C. Furosemide
    D. Reserpin

12. The P wave represents depolarization of the atria. When examining the ECG, you should look for the presence of

    A. P waves in general
    B. a P wave before every QRS complex
    C. a QRS complex before every P wave
    D. all of the above

13. A P-R interval exceeding 0.2 second is called _____ degree AV block.

    A. first
    B. second
    C. third
    D. none of the above

14. Potential causes of sinus tachycardia include

    A. pain and fever
    B. shock and hypoxia
    C. hypotension and congestive heart failure
    D. all of the above

15. The treatment of choice for sinus tachycardia is

    A. atropin sulphate
    B. treatment of the underlying cause
    C. propranolol
    D. all of the above

16. You should NOT treat patients with sinus bradycardia if they have

    A. unconsciousness
    B. a good or strong pulse

C. cold and clammy skin
D. systolic blood pressure of 80 mmHg or less

17. Which of the following drugs can be used to treat sinus bradycardia?

    A. Atropin sulphate
    B. Propranolol
    C. Isoproterenol
    D. A and C *only*

18. For premature atrial contraction,

    A. epinephrine is the best treatment
    B. dopamine is the best treatment
    C. no satisfactory treatment exists
    D. all of the above

19. A 40-year-old male has paroxymal supraventricular tachycardia and stable vital signs. The physician tells you to apply vagal maneuvers but, at the same time, the patient develops hypotension.
    The treatment of choice is

    A. to continue valsalva maneuver
    B. cardioversion
    C. verapamil
    D. digoxin

20. Some maneuvers that stimulate the vagus nerve will slow the heart rate and may convert some PSVT's back to normal sinus rhythm.
    These maneuvers include all of the following EXCEPT

    A. valsalva maneuver
    B. ice water
    C. carotid sinus massage
    D. hot water

21. You are taking a patient with PSVT to the hospital, which is 30 minutes away.
    The physician may tell you to administer

    A. verapamil
    B. digoxin
    C. dopamine
    D. all of the above

22. You are looking at the ECG of a patient who has regular rhythm, a rate of 50 per minute, absent P wave, and normal QRS complexes.
    The MOST likely diagnosis is

    A. sinus bradycardia
    B. junctional bradycardia
    C. third degree heart block
    D. none of the above

23. If the patient in the above question develops signs of poor perfusion, you should administer

    A. atropin sulphate
    B. digoxin
    C. procainamide
    D. all of the above

24. Propranolol is known by the trade name(s)

    A. pronestyle
    B. inderal
    C. procardia
    D. all of the above

Questions 25-30.

DIRECTIONS: In Questions 25 through 30, match the numbered description or function with the appropriate lettered part of the cardiovascular system, as listed in Column I. Place the letter of the CORRECT answer in the space at the right.

COLUMN I
A. Tricuspid valve
B. Mitral valve
C. Coronary sulcus
D. Systole
E. Diastole
F. SA node

25. The groove which separates the atria and the ventricle, in which the arteries and the main coronary vein cross the heart. 25.____

26. Separates the right atrium from the right ventricle. 26.____

27. Separates the left atrium from the left ventricle. 27.____

28. Atrial and ventricular relaxation. 28.____

29. Atrial and ventricular contraction. 29.____

30. Located in the right atrium near the inlet of the superior vena cava. 30.____

KEY (CORRECT ANSWERS)

1. A
2. C
3. C
4. A
5. B

6. D
7. B
8. C
9. D
10. C

11. B
12. D
13. A
14. D
15. B

16. B
17. D
18. C
19. B
20. D

21. A
22. B
23. A
24. B
25. C

26. A
27. B
28. E
29. D
30. F

RESPIRATORY SYSTEM
EXAMINATION SECTION
TEST 1

DIRECTIONS: Each question or incomplete statement is followed by several suggested answers or completions. Select the one that BEST answers the question or completes the statement. *PRINT THE LETTER OF THE CORRECT ANSWER IN THE SPACE AT THE RIGHT.*

1. In the upper respiratory tract,

    A. air is filtered in the nasopharynx
    B. air is warmed to 37° C before reaching the lungs
    C. cilia sweep foreign matter towards the oropharynx where it may be expectorated or swallowed
    D. all of the above

2. The left lung consists of _____ lobe(s).

    A. two
    B. three
    C. one
    D. none of the above

3. Alveoli are NOT

    A. hollow sacs
    B. thick-walled
    C. the agents through which oxygenation occurs
    D. the most important functional unit of the respiratory system

4. By definition, normal ventilation is that which maintains the arterial PCO_2 at APPROXIMATELY _____ to _____ torr.

    A. 10; 15   B. 20; 30   C. 35; 40   D. 50; 60

5. If the arterial PO_2 falls below 80 torr., the patient is considered

    A. hypercapnic
    B. hypocapnic
    C. hyoxemic
    D. tachypnic

6. Elevated PCO_2 is commonly associated with all of the following conditions EXCEPT

    A. myasthenia gravis
    B. stroke
    C. hyperventilation syndrome
    D. head injury

7. Which of the following conditions is(are) associated with hypoxemia?

    A. Near drowning
    B. Pulmonary edema
    C. Chest trauma
    D. All of the above

8. The respiratory control center is located in the part of the brain known as the

   A. medulla
   B. frontal lobe
   C. pineal gland
   D. temporal lobe

9. The one of the following conditions which is NOT a cause of lower airway obstruction is

   A. epiglottitis
   B. emphysema
   C. chronic bronchitis
   D. asthma

10. Causes of respiratory center depression include all of the following EXCEPT

    A. a stroke
    B. pulmonary edema
    C. depressant drugs
    D. head trauma

11. _____ is NOT among the conditions which frequently affect alveoli.

    A. Flail chest
    B. Pneumothorax
    C. Croup
    D. Pulmonary edema

12. Regarding chronic obstructive pulmonary disease, it is FALSE that

    A. the condition is more common among men than women
    B. 82 percent of mortality is attributed to alcohol use
    C. the condition is more common among city dwellers than in rural populations
    D. it is seen primarily in individuals between the ages of 45 and 65

13. All of the following are considered classic features of pink puffers (emphysema) EXCEPT

    A. pain and wasted appearance
    B. barrel-shaped chest which is hyperresonant to percussion owing to air trapping within the lungs
    C. obvious shortness of breath and frequent pursing of the lips during exhalation
    D. none of the above

14. Symptoms and signs of decompensation in COPD include

    A. increasing dyspnea and sleep disturbance
    B. confusion, agitation, and combativeness resulting from hypoxemia
    C. lethargy and drowsiness resulting from hypercarbia
    D. all of the above

15. Of the following, _____ is(are) NOT helpful in the management of COPD.

    A. oxygen by nasal canvia or mask
    B. aminophylline
    C. sedatives and tranquilizers
    D. establishment of an IV lifeline with D5W

16. Among the common clinical features of the acute asthmatic attack is(are)

    A. wheezing that is audible without a stethoscope
    B. spasmodic coughing
    C. prominent use of accessor muscles of respiration
    D. all of the above

17. It is NOT a sign of a severe asthmatic attack when 17._____

    A. pulse rate is greater than 130 per minute
    B. respiratory rate is less than 20 per minute
    C. pulus paradoxus is greater than 15 mmhg
    D. chest is silent

18. Pre-hospital management of an acute asthmatic attack may employ all of the following 18._____
    EXCEPT

    A. albuterol   B. aminophylline
    C. cromolyn sodium   D. epinephrine

19. Of the following statements, which is(are) TRUE regarding bacterial pneumonia? 19._____

    A. Elderly patients with chronic illnesses and smokers are at greater risk to contract the illness.
    B. The most common form of bacterial pnemonia is pneumococcal pneumonia.
    C. The peak incidence occurs in winter and early spring.
    D. All of the above

20. The MOST effective treatment of pneumonia would be the use of 20._____

    A. antibiotics
    B. oxygen
    C. multiple doses of epinephrine
    D. all of the above

21. Specialized respiratory functions include 21._____

    A. coughing or sneezing   B. hiccupping
    C. sighing   D. all of the above

Questions 22-25.

DIRECTIONS: In Questions 22 through 25, match the numbered description with the lettered symptomatic sound it describes listed in Column I. Place the letter of the CORRECT answer in the appropriate space at the right.

COLUMN I

A. Rales
B. Rhonchi
C. Wheezing
D. Stridor

22. Harsh, high-pitched sound upon inspiration indicating an upper airway obstruction. 22._____

23. Harsher sound indicating the presence of fluid in a larger airway. 23._____

24. High-pitched whistling sound of air moving through narrowed airways. 24._____

25. Fine, crackling sound indicating the presence of fluid in a small airway. 25._____

KEY (CORRECT ANSWERS)

1.	D	11.	C
2.	A	12.	B
3.	B	13.	D
4.	C	14.	D
5.	C	15.	C
6.	C	16.	D
7.	D	17.	B
8.	A	18.	C
9.	A	19.	D
10.	B	20.	B

21. D
22. D
23. B
24. C
25. A

TEST 2

DIRECTIONS: Each question or incomplete statement is followed by several suggested answers or completions. Select the one that BEST answers the question or completes the statement. *PRINT THE LETTER OF THE CORRECT ANSWER IN THE SPACE AT THE RIGHT.*

1. Physical factors influencing the respiratory center include all of the following EXCEPT _____ respiratory rate. 1.____

    A. high temperature increasing
    B. low temperature increasing
    C. low blood pressure increasing
    D. high blood pressure decreasing

2. Regarding the effect of carbon dioxide and oxygen on inspiratory activity, it is NOT true that 2.____

    A. high CO_2 concentration decreases respiratory activity
    B. high CO_2 concentration increases respiratory activity
    C. low CO_2 concentration decreases respiratory activity
    D. hypoxemia is the most profound stimulus to respiration in the normal individual

3. The single MOST common cause of airway obstruction in the unconscious victim is due to 3.____

    A. dentures   B. the tongue
    C. a foreign body   D. glottic edema

4. In order to eliminate airway obstruction due to the presence of a foreign body, you should NOT 4.____

    A. discourage the victim from coughing
    B. deliver four blows to the back of the victim
    C. apply abdominal thrust (Heimlich maneuver)
    D. do more than one but not all of the above

5. Among adults, the MOST common factor associated with drowning is 5.____

    A. alcohol intoxication   B. cocaine abuse
    C. heroin intoxication   D. none of the above

6. *A severe prolonged asthmatic attack that cannot be broken with epinephrine* is the definition of 6.____

    A. bronchitis   B. status asthmaticus
    C. asthmatic bronchitis   D. COPD

7. All of the following are true statements regarding near-drowning EXCEPT: 7.____

    A. 10 percent of drowning victims do not aspirate any water at all
    B. The mortality rate from drowning is less than 5 percent
    C. In freshwater drowning, the hypotonic solution has been absorbed through the lungs
    D. In saltwater drowning, pulmonary edema occurs as a result of aspiration

8. Management techniques for cases of near-drowning include

   A. early performance of endotracheal intubation to prevent aspiration
   B. determination of whether the victim has a pulse; if not, starting of external chest compression
   C. insertion of a nasogastric tube to decompress the stomach (only after an endotracheal tube is in place)
   D. all of the above

9. The treatment of choice for severe metabolic acidosis in drowning victims is

   A. hyperventilation by ambu bag
   B. sodium bicarbonate
   C. calcium carbonate
   D. 100% oxygen

10. The one of the following conditions that CANNOT produce pulmonary edema is

    A. heroin overdose
    B. left heart failure
    C. ingestion of furosemide
    D. inhalation of toxic fumes

11. The signs and symptoms of pulmonary edema include all of the following EXCEPT

    A. presence of hypoxia, dyspnea, and cyanosis
    B. patient laboring to breathe, often sitting bolt upright
    C. low arterial CO_2 concentration and high oxygen concentration
    D. rales heard when listening to the posterior bases of both lungs

12. In the management of pulmonary edema, it is NOT necessary to

    A. manage and transport the patient in a sitting position
    B. administer morphine if ordered by a physician
    C. apply rotating tourniquets, if indicated
    D. strictly avoid administering oxygen in high concentration

13. Among the common symptoms of acute mountain sickness is (are) included

    A. throbbing bilateral frontal headache which is worse in the morning and in the supine position
    B. sleep disturbance
    C. dyspnea on exertion
    D. all of the above

14. The MOST useful sign of progression from mild to moderate mountain sickness is

    A. ataxia
    B. lassitude
    C. anorexia
    D. dyspnea on exertion

15. If you anticipate a long delay in arranging rescue for a patient with acute mountain sickness, you should administer

    A. epinephrine
    B. dexamethasone
    C. bronchodilator
    D. none of the above

16. Common signs and symptoms of high altitude pulmonary edema include

    A. tachpnea, severe dysmnea, and chyne-stokes respirations
    B. cough, cyanosis, and tachycardia
    C. confusion and coma
    D. all of the above

17. The MOST important element in treating high altitude pulmonary edema is

    A. descent to lower altitude
    B. intravenous morphine
    C. intravenous diuretics
    D. all of the above

18. _____ are the MOST common scenarios of exposure to toxic gases.

    A. Municipal swimming pools
    B. Fires
    C. Transport accidents
    D. Industrial settings

19. The *dunglung* syndrome of pulmonary edema, metabolic acidosis, and cardiovascular collapse is produced by

    A. hydrogen sulfide
    B. acrylics
    C. cotton
    D. nitrogen dioxide

20. An IMPORTANT part of the treatment of suspected pulmonary embolism is to

    A. ensure an open airway and administer 100% oxygen
    B. monitor cardiac rhythm
    C. establish an IV lifeline with normal saline
    D. all of the above

Questions 21-25.

DIRECTIONS: In Questions 21 through 25, match the numbered characteristic with the lettered disorder listed in Column I with which it is MOST closely associated. Place the letter of the CORRECT answer in the appropriate space at the right.

21. Birth control pill.

22. Patient is often young, thin, and tall.

23. Carpopedal spasms and low CO_2.

24. Extreme obesity, periods of apnea, and dysrhythmias during sleep.

25. Oxygen is the mainstay of treatment.

COLUMN I

A. Pickwickian syndrome
B. Hyperventilation syndrome
C. Chronic obstructive pulmonary disease
D. Pulmonary embolism
E. Spontaneous pneumothorax

KEY (CORRECT ANSWERS)

1. B
2. A
3. B
4. A
5. A

6. B
7. B
8. D
9. B
10. C

11. C
12. D
13. D
14. A
15. B

16. D
17. A
18. B
19. A
20. D

21. D
22. E
23. B
24. A
25. C

CARDIOVASCULAR SYSTEM

TABLE OF CONTENTS

	Page
Unit 1 – Anatomy and Physiology	1
Circulatory System	1
Heart	2
Cardiac Cycle	5
Heart Sounds	6
Cardiac Output	6
Blood Pressure	7
Pulse	7
Nervous Control	7
Electromechanical System of the Heart	9
Physiology of the Specialized Conduction System	9
Cardiac Conduction System	10
Principles of Electrophysiology	11
Unit 2 – Patient Assessment	13
Current Complaint	13
Past Medical History	14
Physical Examination	15
Unit 3 – Pathophysiology and Management of Cardiovascular Problems	18
Coronary Artery Disease and Angina	18
Acute Myocardial Infarction	19
Congestive Heart Failure	22
Cardiogenic Shock	25
Syncope	26
Other Complications of AMI	28
Myocardial Trauma	29
Hypertensive Emergencies	30
Unit 4 – Reading and Understanding a Normal EKG	31
Electrophysiology	31
Components of the EKG Record	32
Reading an EKG Rhythm Strip	32
Unit 5 – Arrhythmia Recognition	35
General Concepts	35
Introduction to Reading Arrhythmias	36
System for Identification of Arrhythmias	38

CARDIOVASCULAR SYSTEM

UNIT 1 – ANATOMY AND PHYSIOLOGY

The cardiovascular system is composed of the heart and blood vessels. The function of the cardiovascular system is to transport blood through the body.

Circulatory System

In the process of circulation, the blood carries certain nutrients (e.g., glucose and proteins) and oxygen to the cells and carries carbon dioxide and metabolic waste products away from them. The blood also carries hormones (e.g., epinephrine) that aid in regulating body processes and antibodies that protect the body from infections.

The vessels that carry blood away from the heart are called arteries. Vessels that return blood to the heart are called veins. The capillaries are blood vessels that connect the arterial and venous systems.

The walls of the arteries and veins are composed of three layers of tissue. The inner layer is called the tunica intima and forms a smooth, thin lining. The middle layer, the tunica media, is the thickest of the three tissue layers. It is composed of elastic tissue and smooth muscle cells that allow the vessels to expand or contract in response to changes in blood pressure and tissue demand. The outer layer of tissue is called the tunica adventitia and consists of elastic and fibrous connective tissue. This layer gives the vessel strength to withstand high blood pressure.

A lumen is a cavity or channel within a tubular organ, the size or diameter of which varies with the size of the organ. The changes in the size of the lumina in the arteries play an important role in regulating blood pressure.

The arteries have thicker walls than the capillaries and veins because they transport blood at higher pressure. The primary function of the large arteries is to conduct blood to smaller arteries called arterioles, which then conduct the blood to capillaries. A second function of the arteries is regulation of blood pressure through changes in peripheral resistance. Since the arterial system functions to deliver blood to the body, there are no valves in the arteries. Approximately 15 percent of the body's blood is contained in the arterial system at any one time.

The arterioles terminate in tiny thin-walled vessels called capillaries. Capillaries are composed of only one layer of tissue called the tunica intima. The lumina of the capillaries are so small that the red blood cells can pass through only in single file, allowing the ready exchange of oxygen, nutrients, and waste products between blood and body cells through the capillary walls.

The network of capillaries (the capillary bed) contains 5 percent of the body's blood. At the end of the capillary beds are the smallest of the veins, called the venules.

The veins, like the arteries, are composed of three tissue layers. Unlike the arteries, however, the walls of the veins are relatively thin, since they carry blood at low pressure. The venules empty into larger veins that flow into still larger veins that ultimately empty into the two major veins of the body, the superior vena cava and the inferior vena cava. Since the pressure in the veins is low, these vessels contain one-way valves that prevent the backflow of blood. Muscular contraction of the extremities aids in the flow of venous blood back to the heart. The venous system contains 80 percent of the body's blood and serves as a blood reservoir.

The circulatory system has two major components—the pulmonary circulation and the systemic circulation. The pulmonary circulation consists of blood that is pumped to the lungs and blood that is returned to the heart. The systemic circulation consists of blood that is pumped to the rest of the body and is returned to the heart.

Although the circulatory system is sometimes considered a "closed" fluid system, there is a large amount of plasma protein lost through the capillary beds into the interstitial spaces. The only way this lost blood can be returned to the circulatory system is through the lymphatic system. The lymphatic capillaries originate in the interstitial space. These capillaries empty into larger lymphatic vessels, have thin walls, and contain valves. Lymph ultimately is emptied into two main vessels, the right lymphatic duct and the thoracic duct. These two ducts empty in the right subclavian and left subclavian veins, respectively. Thus, the lymphatic system assists the venous system by returning the lost protein to the blood.

Heart

The heart is a cone-shaped, hollow, muscular organ located in the mediastinum, the central section of the thorax. The heart is rotated on its side and lies on the diaphragm in front of the trachea and esophagus and between the lungs. The base, or top of the heart, lies behind the sternum at the level of the third rib. The apex, or bottom of the heart, lies at the level of the fifth rib in the left midclavicular line.

Although the size of the heart varies from person to person, on an average it is about 10 to 12 centimeters (cm) long, 9 cm wide, and 6 cm thick. It weighs about 300 grams (g) in males and about 250 g in females. The size of the heart may be visualized as approximately the size of its owner's fist.

The heart is encased in a double-walled sac called the pericardium. Like the pleura, enveloping the lungs, the pericardium is composed of two layers. The outer layer, the parietal pericardium, is in direct contact with the pleura and is attached to the diaphragm and sternum. The inner layer, or visceral pericardium, surrounds the heart. Separating the two pericardial layers is a space filled with pericardial fluid. This fluid acts as a lubricant and allows the heart to contract without producing friction. The pericardium can become inflamed as a result of some disease processes; this situation will produce friction when the heart contracts, causing a pericardial friction rub that can be heard with a stethoscope.

The wall of the heart is composed of three muscle layers: the epicardium, the myocardium, and the endocardium. The epicardium is the outer layer of the heart and is the same as the visceral pericardium. The epicardium consists of elastic fibers and some fat deposits. The middle layer of the heart is called the myocardium. It is the thickest of the three layers, and is composed of cardiac muscle fibers that provide the force that propels the blood. The endocardium is the inner layer of the heart. It is composed of thin connective tissue and forms the inner surface of the heart and the heart valves.

The heart consists of four hollow chambers and two pumping systems. The two atria or upper chambers are located at the base of the heart; the two ventricles are located at the apex. The right and left atria are thin-walled chambers that receive blood returning to the heart. The larger, thick-walled right and left ventricles pump the blood away from the heart. Of the four chambers, the left ventricle has the thickest walls since it is the chamber that pumps blood through the systemic circulation.

The heart can also be thought of as divided into two pumps by a lengthwise wall of muscular tissue called the septum. Each side is composed of one atrium and one ventricle. The part of the septum separating the two atria is called the interatrial septum; the part separating the two ventricles is called the interventricular septum.

The heart chambers are also separated externally. The atria are divided from the ventricles by the atrioventricular groove. The ventricles are separated externally by the anterior and posterior interventricular grooves. The muscle fibers of the two atria are continuous, as are the muscle fibers of the ventricles. It is this external separation that allows the atria and ventricles to contract independently.

The heart is supplied with blood from two main arteries, the coronary arteries. These arteries originate from the base of the ascending aorta immediately above the leaflets or cusps of the aortic valve. The left coronary artery branches off the left cusp of the aorta and travels over and in front of the heart. The left coronary artery bifurcates or divides into two main branches—the anterior descending branch and the circumflex branch.

The left anterior descending branch supplies blood to the left ventricle and the interventricular septum. The left circumflex branch supplies blood to the left atrium and to the lateral wall of the heart.

The right coronary artery branches off the right cusp of the aorta and travels behind the heart where it divides into a posterior descending branch and a right marginal branch. The right coronary artery supplies blood to the right atrium and the right ventricle (see Table 6.1).

TABLE 6.1
Types of Infarction and Complications of Coronary Arteries

Coronary Artery	Major Areas and Structures Supplied
Right coronary artery	SA node (60 percent)
	AV node (90 percent)
	Bundle of His
	Right Atrium and right ventricle
	Inferior surface of left ventricle
	Posterior one-third of septum
Left anterior descending artery	Anterior wall of the left ventricle
	Anterior two-thirds of septum
	Bundle of His
	Right bundle branch
Left circumflex artery	SA node (40 percent)
	AV node (10 percent)
	Lateral wall of left ventricle
	Left atrium

Interconnections (anastomoses) between the coronary arteries are called the coronary collateral vessels. These secondary arteries can enlarge to provide blood to regions of the heart whose blood supply is decreased as a result of an occlusion of one of the main coronary arteries.

The coronary arteries and the veins draining the heart empty into the coronary sinus, a large cardiac vein. This vein, in turn, drains into the right atrium.

The heart has four valves that allow blood to flow in only one direction. These are the tricuspid, mitral, pulmonic, and aortic valves. The two atrioventricular valves, the tricuspid and the mitral valves, are located between the atria and the ventricles. The two semilunar valves, the pulmonic and aortic valves, are located between the ventricles and the major arteries.

The tricuspid valve, named for its three cusps or sections, is located between the right atrium and the right ventricle. The cusps form a ring around the atrioventricular opening, and their free edges project into the ventricle. These free edges are attached to the chordae tendineae, fine tedinous chords of dense connective tissue that attach to papillary muscles in the ventricular wall. The chordae tendiaeae and the papillary muscles prevent the cusps from flopping backward into the atrium, which would result in inadequate functioning of the valve. Blood could then flow from the atrium into the ventricle—in two directions rather than in one.

The mitral valve is located between the left atrium and left ventricle. It is structurally similar to the tricuspid valve, but has only two cusps.

The pulmonic valve is located between the right ventricle and the pulmonary artery. The aortic valve is located between the left ventricle and the aorta. Like the atrioventricular valves, the semilunar valves are composed of dense connective tissue. However, these valves differ structurally from the atrioventricular valves in that each semilunar valve has three pocket-shaped cusps or leaflets. The lower border of each cusp attaches to the arterial wall and the upper borders swing free.

The opening and closing of the valves are regulated by pressure changes in the heart chambers. When the ventricles contract (ventricular systole), the mitral and tricuspid valves close. When the pressure in the ventricles exceeds the pressure in the aorta and pulmonary artery, the pulmonic and aortic valves open. When this process takes place, some of the blood is ejected from the ventricles into the aorta and the pulmonary artery. When the pressure in the ventricles becomes less than the pressure in the aorta and the pulmonary artery, the aortic and pulmonic valves close.

Blood flows continuously into the atria from the great veins. During ventricular systole, blood accumulates in the atria because the atrioventricular valves are closed. After ventricular systole, the ventricles relax (diastole). At this time, the pressure in the atria begins to exceed the pressure in the ventricles causing the mitral and tricuspid valves to open. The blood that has accumulated in the atria rushes into the ventricles, and the cyclic changes in pressures continue.

In summary, during ventricular systole (contraction), the aortic and pulmonic valves are open and the tricuspid and mitral valves are closed. During ventricular diastole (relaxation), the aortic and pulmonic valves are closed and the mitral and tricuspid valves are open. It is important to note that the coronary arteries fill passively during ventricular diastole.

As mentioned earlier, the heart can be considered a two-pump system—a low-pressure pump on the right side and a high-pressure pump on the left side. The right heart pumps blood into the pulmonary circulation; the left heart pumps blood into the systemic circulation.

Unoxygenated blood is returned to the right atrium by three main veins: (1) the superior vena cava that drains unoxygenated blood from the upper part of the body, (2) the inferior vena cams that returns the blood from the lower part of the body, and (3) the coronary sinus that returns the unoxygenated blood from the heart itself.

When the right atrium contracts, the tricuspid valve opens and permits the unoxygenated blood to flow into the right ventricle. The right ventricle then fills with blood. When the right ventricle begins to contract, the tricuspid valve closes and the pulmonic valve opens. This action permits the unoxygenated blood to enter the right and the left pulmonary arteries located at the base of the right ventricle. The blood is then pumped into the lungs. The pulmonary circulation is also known as the "lesser" circulation because less pressure—approximately 30 millimeters of mercury (mm Hg)—is required to pump blood to the lungs than to the rest of the body. The right side of the heart thus functions as a low-pressure pump system.

When the unoxygenated blood reaches the lungs, carbon dioxide leaves the blood and oxygen enters through the capillary bed. The unoxygenated blood then becomes oxygenated. The blood then flows into the pulmonary veins, returns to the heart, and enters the left atrium.

As the left atrium contracts, the mitral valve opens and permits the oxygenated blood to flow into the left ventricle, which then fills with blood. When the left ventricle begins to contract, the mitral valve closes and the aortic valve opens. This action permits the oxygenated blood to enter the aorta, which is located at the base of the left ventricle. Oxygenated blood is then pumped to the rest of the body—head and neck, upper extremities, thorax, digestive tract, liver, kidneys, lower extremities, and the heart itself. This circulation is known as the systemic circulation or "greater" circulation. The amount of pressure that must be generated to pump blood to the rest of the body is quite high, approximately 120 mm Hg. Thus, the left side of the heart functions as a high-pressure pump system.

To review, the oxygenated blood flows through the aorta into the coronary arteries, systemic arteries, arterioles, and capillaries. Oxygen is given up to the tissues, and carbon dioxide and waste products enter the blood at the capillary level. The unoxygenated blood is returned to the heart via the venules and veins, which terminate in the superior and inferior venae cavae. Unoxygenated blood then enters the right atrium and the process continues. Blood is never directly exchanged between the right and left sides of the heart.

Cardiac Cycle

Although each side of the heart may be considered as a separate pump, both sides, in fact, work in parallel. That is, both atria contract simultaneously, followed by both ventricles. The actual time sequence between ventricular contraction (systole) and relaxation (diastole) is called the cardiac cycle.

As previously described, during ventricular diastole, the ventricles fill passively with 70 percent of the blood that has accumulated in the atria. Active contraction of the atria forces the remaining 30 percent of the blood into the ventricles. Atrial contraction plays only a small part in ventricular filling. Therefore, if the atria do not contract, ventricular filling still occurs. The volume of blood in the ventricles at the end of the diastole is normally 100 to 150 milliliters (ml).

Systole lasts about 0.28 second; diastole, about 0.52 second. Therefore, one cardiac cycle occurs every 0.8 second. At faster heart rates the time for diastole decreases, while the time for systole remains virtually unchanged. Consequently, ventricular filling decreases with fast heart rates.

Heart Sounds

Closure of the heart valves during the cardiac cycle produces two heart sounds. These sounds result from movement of blood when the valves close. Closure of the mitral and tricuspid valves at the beginning of systole produces the first heart sound ("lub"). The second sound ("dub") occurs with the closure of the aortic and pulmonary valves at the beginning of diastole.

Cardiac Output

Cardiac work is measured by the amount of blood the heart pumps each minute (cardiac output). Since the ventricles contract simultaneously, their outputs are normally equal. Cardiac output (CO) equals stroke volume (SV) multiplied by heart rate (HR).

Stroke volume is the amount of blood pumped by either ventricle during one cardiac cycle or heart beat. Heart rate is the number of contractions, or beats, per minute. Stroke volume is normally 60 to 100 ml per beat; the heart rate is usually 60 to 100 beats per minute. Using SV and HR, the paramedic can determine the cardiac output. Therefore, if a person has an SV of 70 ml per beat and an HR of 70 beats per minute, the cardiac output will be approximately 5 liters per minute.

70 ml per beat X 70 beats per minute = 490 ml per minute

or

approximately 5 l per minute

Any change in heart rate or stroke volume will effect a change in the cardiac output. For example, an increase in either heart rate or stroke volume will increase the cardiac output.

Stroke volume is the amount of blood pumped by the ventricles with each contraction. An increase in volume in the ventricles causes a more forceful contraction stretching the ventricular myocardial fibers resulting in a more forceful contraction. This principle is referred to as Starling's law. Therefore, using the formula CO = SV X HR, it can be seen that if stroke volume increases but heart rate remains constant, cardiac output will increase. However, if the myocardial muscle fibers are continuously stretched, they lose this responsiveness and contract less forcefully than normal. When this happens, cardiac output will no longer be increased by greater stroke volume.

From the equation CO = SV X HR, it is evident that any change in the heart rate will also affect cardiac output. Normally stroke volume is decreased by rapid heart rates. Theoretically, if stroke volume remains constant, cardiac output will be increased by an increase in heart rate.

Blood Pressure

Arterial blood pressure changes during the cardiac cycle. The higher pressure that is reached during ventricular systole is the systolic blood pressure; the lower pressure, reached during ventricular diastole, is the diastolic blood pressure. The difference between the systolic and diastolic blood pressure is called the pulse pressure.

Blood pressure (BP) is related to cardiac output and peripheral vascular resistance (PVR). Peripheral vascular resistance refers to the amount of opposition to blood flow offered by the arterioles. Peripheral vascular resistance is determined by arteriole vasoconstriction and vasodilation. The interrelationships between the EP, CO, and PVR are major factors in maintaining adequate tissue perfusion. This interrelationship can be expressed in the following formula:

$$BP = CO \times PVR$$

If cardiac output or peripheral vascular resistance changes, blood pressure will also change.

Blood pressure will increase or decrease if cardiac output increases or decreases, provided that peripheral vascular resistance remains constant.

If cardiac output remains constant, blood pressure will increase or decrease in response to changes in peripheral vascular resistance. If the arterioles dilate, peripheral vascular resistance to blood flow will be decreased and blood pressure will decrease. With vasoconstrictions, there is an increase in resistance to flow; thus, blood pressure will increase.

Pulse

The pulsation palpated with the fingertips over an artery represents the expansion and recoil of the elastic arterial wall and also gives a measure of the heart rate. With ventricular contraction, the ejected blood expands the walls of the aorta and is transmitted as a pressure wave. This pressure wave cannot be felt in the veins or capillaries because it has been damped out by the time it reaches these vessels.

The pulse should be described according to its rate (fast or slow), its strength (weak and thready; strong and bounding), and its rhythm (regular or irregular).

Nervous Control

The autonomic nervous system regulates the activity of the visceral organs and the blood vessels. The autonomic nervous system also assists the body in adapting to changing physiological conditions. There are two divisions of the autonomic nervous system—the sympathetic nervous system and the parasympathetic nervous system. Almost all the organs of the body are innervated by both divisions; however, each division is antagonistic in action to the other.

The sympathetic nervous system has two types of receptor fibers at its nerve endings—the alpha receptors and the beta receptors. When the sympathetic nervous system is stimulated, norepinephrine is released to transmit the impulse at the nerve ending. Nerve endings that secrete norepinephrine are called adrenergic. When the parasympathetic nervous system is stimulated, acetylcholine is released. When acetylcholine is secreted, the nerve ending is referred to as cholinergic. There are also a few sympathetic nerve fibers that release acetylcholine.

All the blood vessels, except capillaries, have alpha-adrenergic receptors. When these receptors are stimulated, vasoconstriction occurs. The heart and lungs have beta-adrenergic receptors. When they are stimulated, the heart rate increases and the bronchioles dilate.

Blood flow may be regulated either by the autonomic nervous system or by internal hormonal mechanisms such as epinephrine. Because the heart and brain are very sensitive to hypoxia, blood flow to these two organs is regulated mainly by internal mechanisms or changes in oxygen pressure (PO_2) or carbon dioxide pressure (PCO_2). Cerebral and coronary arterioles dilate in response to either decreased PO_2 or increased PCO_2.

Pulmonary blood flow is also regulated mainly by changes in PO_2 or PCO_2. Pulmonary blood vessels, however, constrict in response to decreased PO_2 or increased PCO_2. This response will shunt blood to better ventilated alveoli where carbon dioxide and oxygen exchange can occur.

Blood flow through the skin, kidneys, visceral organs, and skeletal muscle is regulated mainly by the sympathetic nervous system. Arterioles in the skin, kidneys, and visceral organs contain mostly alpha receptors. When alpha receptors are stimulated, these arterioles constrict, and blood flow through the skin, kidneys, and visceral organs is reduced. In arterioles contained in skeletal muscle, beta-adrenergic receptors predominate. These arterioles dilate in response to sympathetic nervous stimulation, which increases blood flow through skeletal muscle.

Blood pressure equals total peripheral resistance times cardiac output, thus, changes in either cardiac output or arteriolar resistance alter blood pressure. The cardiovascular centers in the brain stem control blood pressure. These centers receive messages from pressure receptors in the aortic arch and the carotid sinuses. These pressure receptors fire more rapidly when the arterial blood pressure increases. The cardiovascular centers respond to these rapid firing rates and stimulate the parasympathetic nervous system causing a slowing of the heart rate and a decrease in myocardial contractility; this in turn results in a fall in cardiac output. In addition, decreased stimulation of alpha- and beta-adrenergic receptors reduces arteriolar vasoconstriction and results in a decrease in total peripheral resistance. These two effects, decreased cardiac output and decreased peripheral resistance, combine to reduce the blood pressure toward normal.

In contrast, when the blood pressure falls, fewer messages from the pressure receptors reach the cardiovascular centers. Therefore, the cardiovascular centers increase sympathetic stimulation to the heart and blood vessels and decrease parasympathetic stimulation. Sympathetic stimulation of the beta receptors in the heart increases contractility of the ventricles. Decreased parasympathetic stimulation, likewise, increases the heart rate, thus increasing cardiac output. Arterioles in the skin, kidneys, and visceral organs constrict in response to alpha-adrenergic stimulation. The net effect is increased total peripheral resistance. These three effects, increased contractility, increased heart rate, and increased peripheral resistance, combine to return the blood pressure toward normal.

Hypoxia and carbon dioxide retention also influence blood pressure regulation by the autonomic nervous system. Peripheral chemoreceptors in the aortic and carotid bodies are stimulated by decreased PCO_2, decreased pH, and increased PO_2. Messages from these chemoreceptors reach the cardiovascular centers, which then increase heart rate, force of cardiac contraction, and peripheral resistance. Blood pressure, therefore, rises.

Electromechanical System of the Heart

The heart has a specialized electrical conduction system that is composed of specialized noncontractile tissue. This electrical network serves to coordinate the contraction of the atria and the ventricles. The electrical conduction system includes the sinoatrial (SA) node, the atrial internodal pathways, the atrioventricular (AV) node within the AV junction, the common bundle of His, the right and left bundle branches, and the Purkinje network consisting of Purkinje fibers and their branches.

The SA node is located at the junction of the superior vena cava and the right atrium. The SA node is normally the dominant pacemaker of the heart. Three atrial internodal pathways transmit the electrical impulse from the SA node to the AV node. The AV node is located on the right side of the interatrial septum just above the coronary sinus opening. The AV node serves to slow the impulses from the SA node to the ventricles. From the AV node, conduction resumes its rapid velocity in the bundle of His. The bundle of His then divides into the right and left bundle branches. These branches terminate in Purkinje fibers.

Like all other organs, the heart is innervated by both sympathetic and parasympathetic nerve fibers. The heart has only beta-adrenergic receptors located in the atria and ventricles. Thus, all sympathetic nervous system effects on the heart are beta-adrenergic effects. When the sympathetic nervous system is stimulated, there is an increase in heart rate and contractility. The parasympathetic nervous system acts on the heart via the vagus nerve. Vagal nerve fibers innervate the SA node, atrial muscle, and the AV node. Stimulation of the parasympathetic nervous system will result in slowing of the heart rate and conduction through the AV node, as well as a decrease in atrial contractility.

Physiology of the Specialized Conduction System

All atrial muscle cells contract simultaneously; similarly, all ventricular muscle cells contract together. If a stimulus is strong enough for cardiac cells to reach threshold, all cells will respond to the stimulus and contract. (Threshold is the point at which a stimulus will cause the cell to respond.) This phenomenon is called the "all or none" theory of cardiac muscle cells—all cells will respond or none will. Cardiac muscle cells can contract in response to thermal, electrical, chemical, or mechanical stimuli.

Cardiac muscle cells have the special properties of irritability, conductivity, rhythmicity, and autoinaticity. Rhythmicity is the coordination of the contractions of the cardiac muscle cells to produce a regular heart beat. Automaticity is the ability of cardiac cells to depolarize spontaneously without nervous stimulation. Each group of cardiac cells has an intrinsic or characteristic spontaneous depolarization frequency. When the heart muscle cells depolarize, they normally contract. Therefore, automaticity permits cardiac muscle cells to contract spontaneously without nervous stimulation.

All living cells are surrounded by a semipermeable membrane that serves to maintain the integrity of the cell. The composition of the intracellular compartment differs from that of the extracellular compartment. Potassium is the major intracellular electrolyte. There is 30 times more potassium inside the cell than outside the cell. Sodium is the major extracellular electrolyte. There is 30 times more sodium outside the cell, than inside.

As a result of this variation in electrolyte concentration, the interior of the cell is considered to be electronegative, and the exterior is electropositive. This electrical difference must exist in order for the cell to contract (to produce work). When stimulated, the semipermeable membrane becomes more permeable to sodium. This increased permeability results in an influx of positive ions to the intracellular compartment and a flow of negative ions into the extracellular compartment.

The cell at rest is electronegative and retains potassium. Likewise, the exterior of the cell remains electropositive and sodium is kept out of the cell. The cell at rest is said to be polarized.

When a stimulus of sufficient strength causes the cell to reach threshold, depolarization begins. Not all cells, however, respond at the same threshold. When stimulated, the cell membrane becomes more permeable to sodium. When stimulation occurs, sodium begins to rush into the electronegative cell, reversing the membrane potential; the inside of the cell then becomes electropositive. This rapid change in electrical potential from negative to positive is called depolarization. The wave of depolarization moves across the cells causing the cell to produce work.

After contracting, the cell returns to its resting state through the process of repolarization. The cell membrane contains a "pump" that actively ejects sodium from the intracellular compartment back into the extracellular compartment. The inside of the cell returns to its original electronegative state. The cell is again polarized and can be stimulated again.

During most of repolarization, the cell cannot respond to any new electrical stimulus nor can it spontaneously depolarize. This phase is called the absolute refractory period of the cell. During the relative refractory period, repolarization is almost complete, and the cell can be stimulated to contract prematurely. However, the stimulus must be stronger than normal. At the end of the repolarization period, the cell becomes very sensitive and can be stimulated by minimal stimuli. Stimulation at the end of the repolarization period will result in loss of effective contraction. This phase of repolarization is identified as the vulnerable period of the cell.

Automaticity of cardiac cells depends on normal extracellular electrolyte concentrations. Normal concentrations of potassium, calcium, and sodium are especially important in maintaining automaticity. Increases in the serum concentrations of these electrolytes increase the level of threshold. Thus, automaticity is decreased. Decreases in serum potassium and calcium decrease the threshold level, thus, also increasing automaticity.

Cardiac Conduction System

Each component of the conduction system has a characteristic or intrinsic spontaneous depolarization rate. The SA node depolarizes at a rate of 60 to 100 times per minute; the AV node depolarizes 40 to 60 times per minute; and the bundle branches, at a rate of 20 to 40 times per minute. The SA node normally is the pacemaker of the heart because it reaches threshold first. The wave of depolarization generated by the SA node reaches and stimulates the other cardiac cells before they themselves can depolarize spontaneously. Any area of the heart can become the pacemaker if its depolarization rate becomes faster than the rates of other areas, or if the faster areas fail to depolarize.

From the SA node, the wave of depolarization spreads through the atrial muscle and causes the atria to contract, producing atrial systole. Because the atrial and ventricular muscles are separated, impulses from the atrial muscles do not reach the ventricles. Therefore, three atrial internodal pathways carry the electrical impulse from the SA node to the AV node. It takes approximately 0.08 second for the impulse to travel from the SA node to the AV node. The impulse travels through the AV node relatively slowly. This allows the ventricle to fill with blood.

From the AV node, the impulse travels to the bundle of His. From the bundle of His, the impulse is conducted to the right and left bundle branches that, in turn, conduct the impulse to the Purkinje fibers. It takes approximately 0.10 second for the electrical impulse to be conducted through the ventricles. When the Purkinje fibers are stimulated, the ventricles contract.

Principles of Electrophysiology

Atrial and ventricular depolarization are electrical events that can be sensed by electrodes on the skin surface. If the electrical impulses that reach the electrodes are amplified, they can be recorded in the form of an electrocardiogram (EKG). The EKG is, therefore, a graphic tracing of the electrical activity of the heart, but not the mechanical activity; the EKG does not show how well the heart is contracting.

Any wave or complex of waves recorded on the ERG can be referred to as a positive deflection (above the isoelectric baseline) or as a negative deflection (below the isoelectric baseline). A wave of positive charges moving toward a positive electrode will produce a positive deflection or a deflection above the isoelectric baseline on the ERG. If a wave of positive charges moves away from a positive electrode, a downward or negative deflection will be produced below the baseline. The same electrical event in the heart may produce either a positive or negative deflection on the ERG depending on the position of the positive electrode.

In the following discussion, the components of the ERG as they appear in limb leads I and II will be examined. Electrode placement for these leads is described in the techniques section of this chapter.

During a normal cardiac cycle, the SA node fires first and sends an electrical impulse to stimulate both atria. This produces the P wave, a smoothly rounded upward deflection, which is about 0.10 second long. The P wave represents atrial depolarization.

The impulse then reaches the AV node where there is an 0.08 to 0.16-second pause while the impulse travels through the AV node. This allows the ventricles to fill with blood before contracting.

After the pause at the AV node, the electrical impulse is conducted to the bundle of His. From the bundle of His, the impulse travels through the right and left bundle branches, to the Purkinje fibers, and, ultimately, to the ventricular muscle cells. This produces the QRS complex: The QRS complex consists of the Q, R, and S waves. The Q wave is the first downward deflection of the QRS complex. The first upward deflection of the QRS complex is the R wave. The R wave is the largest deflection in leads I and II. Following the R wave, there is a downward deflection, which is the S wave. The QRS complex, thus, represents ventricular depolarization.

After ventricular depolarization, there is a pause shown by the S-T segment. The S-T segment represents the time during which the ventricles are depolarized and ventricular repolarization can begin again. The S-T segment is usually isoelectric, that is, even with the baseline. The T wave, which represents ventricular repolarization, follows the S-T segment. Ventricular repolarization is strictly an electrical event; there is no associated ventricular movement. In leads I and II, the T wave is normally a slightly asymmetrical, slightly rounded, positive deflection.

In summary:

- The P wave represents atrial depolarization.
- The QRS complex represents ventricular depolarization.
- The T wave represents ventricular repolarization.

An atrial T wave representing repolarization also follows the P wave. However, it usually is not visible on the ERG because it is buried in the QRS complex. The P-QRS-T pattern represents one cardiac cycle.

Segments and intervals are also identified on the EKG. A segment is a section of the EKG between waves; an interval is a section of the EKG that usually contains a wave. The S-T segment represents the time from the end of the S wave to the beginning of the T wave. The P-R interval represents the time from the beginning of the P wave to the beginning of the QRS complex. The normal P-R interval ranges from 0.12 to 0.20 second. The R-R interval represents the time interval between two successive QRS complexes. This will be discussed in more detail in Unit 4.

UNIT 2 – PATIENT ASSESSMENT

The patient with suspected cardiac disease needs to have as complete a history as possible taken and a physical examination given to provide proper preventive care or emergency intervention if necessary. It is important for the paramedic to remember that other body systems may affect, or may be affected by, the cardiac disease process.

Current Complaint

Much information regarding the patient's cardiac problem can be gained from the patient's medical history. The most common chief complaints found in patients suffering from cardiac disease are chest pain, dyspnea, fainting, and palpitations.

Chest pain is often the presenting sign of myocardial infarction. However, other descriptive factors need to be obtained to characterize the patient's condition. These descriptions include the location of the pain, radiation, onset, duration, severity, alleviating factors, aggravating factors, and associated symptoms.

The anatomical location of the pain must be determined. (Does the pain radiate? Does the pain travel to the jaw, down the left arm, into the back?) Onset refers to the time and setting in which the pain first occurred. The onset of chest pain may be sudden or gradual, and it can be precipitated in a variety of settings (after shoveling snow, at rest). Duration refers to the length of time the pain lasts. Severity depends on the subjective analysis of the pain by the patient (feeling of impending doom, squeezing, burning). There may be associated symptoms that also reflect the presence of a cardiac problem (nausea, vomiting, weakness, fatigue). Factors that influence the chest pain include those that aggravate or alleviate the chest pain, as well as medications the patient may have taken to relieve the pain. Finally, it is important to know if the patient has ever experienced this type of pain before, and if so, whether the precipitating factors, the duration, and the severity were the same as in the past. If the patient has a history of chest pain, it is imperative to determine the differences (if any) in the patient's present complaint of chest pain.

Dyspnea, or difficulty in breathing, is another common manifestation of a cardiac problem. Dyspnea may indicate congestive heart failure. As in chest pain, descriptive factors need to be obtained to characterize the patient's condition. These factors include the onset, duration, severity, aggravating factors, alleviating factors, associated symptoms, and prior occurrence.

Onset and duration refer to when and how long the dyspnea occurred. (Did it wake the patient from sleep?) Paroxysmal nocturnal dyspnea (PND) is an acute episode of dyspnea in which the patient suddenly wakes from sleep with a feeling of suffocation. Factors that influence dyspnea include those that alleviate or aggravate the condition—such as changes in body position. Dyspnea that worsens when the patient lies down is referred to as orthopnea and is due to pooling of blood in the lungs when the body is horizontal. Frequently, patients with orthopnea will sleep on several pillows to obtain an upright or semiupright position to avoid further exacerbations of dyspnea. Associated symptoms such as a cough or going to a window to breathe may also be present. It is also important for the paramedic to know if the patient has ever experienced this type of dyspnea before and, if so, whether the circumstances differed from those in the present situation. Dyspnea can result from lung disease as well as heart disease. Therefore, the possibility of an existing chronic pulmonary problem as a cause of the present complaint should also be considered.

Syncope, or fainting, occurs when cardiac output is reduced resulting in inadequate cerebral perfusion. Syncope may be due to cardiac arrhythmias, increased vagal tone, or various heart lesions. It must be determined under what circumstances the syncopal episode occurred and whether the episode was preceded by any warning. It is important that the paramedic know the position the patient was in at the time of the syncopal episode (standing, sitting, lying down). Associated symptoms that may characterize the syncopal episode, such as vomiting, urinary incontinence, or seizure activity, should also be noted. Finally, it is essential that the paramedic know if the patient has ever experienced fainting episodes before arid, if so, if the circumstances were similar.

Palpitations are an abnormal awareness of one's heartbeat. Palpitations can result from a cardiac arrhythmia, such as premature systole or paroxysmal tachycardia. Patients may describe palpitations by saying their hearts have "skipped a beat." Palpitations can also be associated with exercise, stimulants such as caffeine, and metabolic disturbances such as hyperthyroidism. It is important for the paramedic to determine onset, frequency, duration, previous episodes of palpitations, and the type of sensation the patient experiences, such as rapid beating, irregular beating, or forceful beating. Associated symptoms such as chest pain, dyspnea, or syncope also can be present.

Past Medical History

After exploring the nature of the present illness, the paramedic should explore pertinent aspects of the patient's past medical history that may contribute to defining the problem. Four major factors should be considered when taking a past medical history: (1) current medications, (2) any present serious illness, (3) presence of cardiac risk factors, and (4) allergies.

It is important that the paramedic note all the medications a patient is taking, especially those medications that might contribute to defining the current problem. The paramedic should particularly note whether the patient takes any of the following medications:

- Nitroglycerin, a drug to relieve chest pain
- Digitalis, a preparation such as digoxin that is often prescribed for congestive heart failure
- Diuretic, a medication such as furosemide (Lasix), commonly prescribed for hypertension or congestive heart failure
- Procainamide or quinidine, drugs that suppress chronic arrhythmias
- Propranolol, a drug prescribed to relieve chest pain or to suppress chronic arrhythmias

Is the patient currently under treatment for any serious illness, such as an infectious disease? Has the patient ever had any illnesses that are considered as cardiac risk factors? These conditions include hypertension, diabetes, previous heart attack or heart failure, rheumatic fever, or lung disease.

Does the patient have any allergies, especially drug allergies such as to Novocain? (Novocain is the numbing medication used in the dentist's office.) Novocain is related to lidocaine. Patients who have had an adverse reaction to Novocain may likewise have a reaction to lidocaine. It is essential to know if the patient is allergic to Novocain in case the patient develops arrhythmias that might necessitate the use of lidocaine.

Physical Examination

The primary and secondary surveys of cardiac patients are similar to those for all patients. Certain parts of the physical examination, however, are emphasized in the patient with heart problems. The physical findings are then correlated with the patient history to evaluate the current complaint.

As in the physical examination of every patient, the paramedic should first take the vital signs. A blood pressure reading over 140/90 indicates hypertension; however, in emergency situations, an elevated blood pressure may be due to anxiety. A systolic blood pressure of less than 90 mm Hg is usually an indication of serious hypotension and shock. The rate and quality of the pulse may give important clues to the critical nature of the patient's problem. Tachycardia may indicate anxiety, pain, congestive heart failure, or cardiac arrhythmia.

Pulse pressure (the difference between the systolic pressure and diastolic pressure) indicates both stroke volume and arterial elasticity. In arteriosclerosis (hardening of the arteries), the arteries are more rigid and the pulse pressure is increased. In cardiogenic shock, the heart is unable to pump a normal stroke volume resulting in a fall in pulse pressure.

The patient's state of consciousness should also be checked as it indicates the adequacy of cerebral perfusion. Stupor or confusion often indicates inadequate cardiac output, which causes a reduction in cerebral perfusion. Skin color and temperature are important indicators of peripheral perfusion. The cold, sweaty skin of many patients with myocardial infarction signifies massive peripheral vasoconstriction.

The status of the patient's external jugular veins should also be checked during the head-to-toe survey. The neck veins provide an estimate of venous pressure in lieu of a central venous pressure line. Normally, when a patient is sitting or standing, the external jugular veins are collapsed above the suprasternal notch. Therefore, when a patient is sitting at a 450 angle, venous distention is not normally present. Elevated venous pressure is associated with congestive (right) heart failure, pericardial tamponade, tricuspid stenosis, and increased blood volume.

To estimate venous pressure, the paramedic should place the patient in a semisitting position at an angle of between 300 and 60° (usually at a 450 angle) with the head slightly rotated away from the external jugular vein being examined. The examiner should place the forefinger just above, and parallel to, the clavicle. The paramedic should place a finger inward to occlude the jugular vein, and wait 15 to 45 seconds for the vein to fill and become distended. The finger should then be quickly released and the height of the distended fluid column within the vein observed. Normally, this level, if visible, will be less than 3 cm above the sternal angle. When reporting the amount of neck vein distention, it is important that the paramedic relates at what angle the patient was sitting.

The lungs must be auscultated for the presence of tales or wheezes that, if present, may indicate pulmonary edema as a result of left heart failure.

To examine the heart, it is helpful for the paramedic to recall the location of the heart chambers and great vessels relative to the chest wall. The apex of the heart is in the fifth intercostal space slightly medial to the center of the clavicle; the base of the heart is at the level of the third costal cartilages. The inferior surface of the heart lies on the diaphragm.

Most of the anterior surface of the heart is formed by the right ventricle. The left ventricle lies to the left and behind the right ventricle. The right border of the heart is formed by the right atrium. The ascending aorta lies behind the sternum from the second through the fourth costal cartilages. The pulmonary artery lies slightly to the left of the ascending aorta; the superior vena cava lies to the right.

A complete examination of the heart is not adaptable to field use. Many such findings are esoteric and often paramedics do not have the proper equipment or must work in surroundings not conducive to performing a complete cardiac examination of inspection, palpation, and auscultation.

Abnormal vibrations from a diseased aortic valve and pulsations from an aortic aneurysm can be detected by palpation of the aortic area located in the second intercostal space to the right of the sternum. Pulmonary artery pulsations can be detected in the pulmonic area located in the second intercostal space to the left of the sternum. Left ventricular contraction normally produces a visible and palpable impulse at the apex located in the fifth intercostal space, medial to the left midclavicular line.

To auscultate the heart, both the diaphragm and bell of the stethoscope should be used. The environment must be as quiet as possible for auscultation to be done correctly. However, since a more sophisticated cardiac auscultation can be conducted under more favorable conditions in the hospital, only a general discussion of heart sounds follows.

Prior to listening for heart sounds, the paramedic should identify the heart rate and heart rhythm at the apex. Since the apical pulse represents the contraction of the left ventricle, it is the best source for determining heart rate. Normally, the apical pulse is the same as the radial pulse. However, if the patient has a tachyarrhythmia, there may be a difference between the radial and apical pulse. This is known as pulse deficit.

Heart sounds are produced by the closure of the heart valves during a cardiac cycle. Audibility of heart sounds varies with the position of the stethoscope and the size of the chest wall. Heart sounds may be inaudible in obese, heavy-chested individuals, and quite loud in thin-chested patients.

Four main topographic areas are used in cardiac auscultation—the aortic, pulmonic, and apical (also called mitral) areas, as described above, as well as the tricuspid area, which is in the fifth intercostal space at the left of the sternum. These areas do not correspond to the anatomic locations of the valves, but are sites at which the particular valve is heard best.

The first heart sound (S_1) is the systole, or "lub," and represents the closure of the mitral and tricuspid valves. The second heart sound (S_2), or "dub," is the diastole and represents the closure of the aortic and pulmonic valves. Normally, diastole is longer than systole.

Sometimes, a third heart sound (S_3) may be heard approximately one-third through diastole and will produce a rhythm that sounds like:

"Ken - tuc' - ky,   Ken - tuc' - ky"
(S_1) - (S_2) - (S_3)   (S_1) - (S_2) - (S_3)

A third heart sound is normal in children and young adults before age 30. Beyond age of 30, an S_3 often indicates the presence of congestive heart failure. If, during auscultation of the lungs, rales or wheezes are heard, auscultation of the heart for the presence of an S_3 could aid in confirming the finding of congestive heart failure.

If a suspected cardiac patient presents with signs of congestive heart failure--rales, distended neck veins, and/or an S_3—the lower back (sacrum) and the legs should also be checked for the presence of edema.

To evaluate the integrity of the vascular system, the carotid, brachial, radial, femoral, popliteal, and dorsalis pedis pulses should be palpated. The strength of these pulses should be noted as well as whether they are equal on both sides. An absent pulse at any one of these sites may indicate that the patient is severely hypotensive, or that the artery is occluded.

If the patient is not hypotensive and one of the pulses cannot be palpated, the extremity must be checked for signs of arterial occlusion. Classic signs of arterial occlusion are the "5 P's": pain, paralysis, paresthesia (an abnormal sensation as burning, prickling, or numbness), pulselessness, and pallor. In 50 percent of these patients, pain is not the presenting symptom, but the extremity will feel cold and/or numb to the touch. The extremity will also appear pale or cyanotic. The pulse is absent or diminished in strength below the level of occlusion. Without treatment, 50 percent of these patients will develop gangrene, which will necessitate amputation of the affected extremity. Approximately 40 percent of these patients will die if sudden arterial occlusion is left untreated.

UNIT 3 – PATHOPHYSIOLOGY AND MANAGEMENT OF CARDIOVASCULAR PROBLEMS

The pathophysiology and management of eight cardiovascular problems are discussed in this section. These problems include coronary artery disease, angina, acute myocardial infarction, congestive heart failure, cardiogenic shock, syncope, myocardial trauma, and hypertensive emergencies.

Coronary Artery Disease and Angina

The coronary arteries are blood vessels that supply the heart with nutrients and oxygen. When a coronary artery becomes blocked, the heart muscle it supplies is rapidly deprived of oxygen. If oxygen deprivation remains uncorrected, the heart muscle will die.

Arteriosclerosis is a degenerative disease that hardens and narrows arteries. A common type of arteriosclerosis, intimal atherosclerosis, is particularly important because it involves the aorta and the cerebral and coronary arteries. Coronary arteries are especially prone to atherosclerosis. Turbulent blood flow and numerous bends contribute to thickening and loss of elasticity in the arterial walls. These conditions result in narrowing of the arteries and a reduction in arterial blood flow.

Approximately 4 to 5 million Americans have coronary artery disease, and more than half a million of these die each year from it.

Certain factors increase an individual's risk of developing atherosclerotic lesions that will lead to coronary artery disease. These risk factors include:

- Hypertension
- Cigarette smoking
- Diabetes
- Elevated serum cholesterol
- Sedentary lifestyle
- Dietary habits (excessive intake of calories, carbohydrates, and/or saturated fats)
- Obesity
- Sex (male)
- Family history
- Aggressive, competitive personality (so-called type-A personality)
- Stressful occupation or environment
- Use of birth control pills

Atherosclerosis is a gradual process involving obstruction and hardening of the arterial wall. In the beginning, small cholesterol and lipid (fat) deposits form on the intima, usually in an area where platelets have attached or a blood clot was formed. These deposits enlarge and irritate the arterial wall. The artery reacts to this irritation by swelling and growing new capillaries. Scar formation (fibrosis) follows and a calcification process begins. During the inflammatory state, capillaries may rupture and bleed into the arterial wall. This produces blood clots, which further narrow the lumen and critically reduce arterial blood flow. Eventually, the intima becomes thickened, hardened, and inelastic.

As portions of a coronary artery become obstructed, other vascular pathways enlarge. These vascular pathways are identified as the collateral coronary circulation. The collateral arteries serve as an alternative route for blood flow around the obstructed artery to the myocardium.

Patients in the early stages of atherosclerosis may be asymptomatic and may continue so for many years. However, when atherosclerosis has progressed to the point that coronary blood flow can no longer meet the oxygen demands of the myocardium, pain will result. The principal symptom of coronary artery disease is angina pectoris, which literally means "choking in the chest." Angina occurs when there is a discrepancy between the oxygen requirements and the oxygen supply to the myocardium. The myocardium, consequently, becomes ischemic, and lactic acid and carbon dioxide accumulate. The concept of supply and demand is important in this context. The individual at rest may have an adequate supply of oxygen to the heart in spite of narrowed coronary arteries; however, when the individual exercises or experiences some other physical or emotional stress, blood flow to the heart cannot meet its increased oxygen demand, and angina results. The patient who experiences angina at rest, when oxygen needs are minimal, has much more severe coronary artery disease than the patient who experiences angina only with vigorous exercise.

Angina pectoris is variable in its presentation, but is classically characterized as substernal chest pain that may be pressing, tight, or squeezing. Anginal pain may radiate to either shoulder and arm, but most commonly radiates to the left shoulder and the left arm. Pain may also radiate to the neck, jaw and teeth, upper back, or epigastrium. Angina is not influenced by respiration, coughing, or changes in body movement. Angina usually lasts 3 to 5 minutes and is transient in nature. The condition can be relieved by stopping the precipitating stress factor or through use of the drug nitroglycerin. Nitroglycerin acts by causing peripheral vasodilation, which reduces myocardial workload and myocardial oxygen demand.

It is important for the paramedic to distinguish between stable and unstable angina. Stable angina follows a recurrent, predictable pattern. The individual experiences pain after a certain amount of physical exertion, such as climbing a flight of stairs, or after situations with some amount of emotional impact. The pain produced also has a predictable location, intensity, and duration. The patient with stable angina may state, "Every time I walk to the bus stop, I get a squeezing pain under my breastbone and I have to sit down for 2 or 3 minutes until it goes away."

Unstable angina ("preinfarction angina") is much more ominous than stable angina, and indicates further coronary artery obstruction.

Unstable angina is characterized by a change in the frequency, intensity, and/or duration of the pain and often occurs without a precipitating stress. The patient may state that over the past several days or weeks the anginal attacks have grown more frequent or more severe, or that they occur during rest. Unstable angina is a warning of impending myocardial infarction.

Acute Myocardial Infarction

Acute myocardial infarction (AMI) ("heart attack") occurs when part of the cardiac muscle is deprived of an adequate supply of blood long enough that the muscle dies (necrosis). Many factors can acutely decrease flow through coronary vessels already narrowed by atherosclerosis.

The precipitating factors of any acute myocardial infarction include occlusion of a coronary artery by a blood clot (thrombus) and conditions that reduce blood flow throughout the body (shock, dysrhythmias, pulmonary embolism, etc.).

AMI is the leading cause of death in the United States today. There are more than half a million deaths from AMI in this country each year. Of those deaths, more than half occur during the first 2 to 3 hours outside the hospital. Ninety percent of deaths from AMI are caused by arrhythmias, usually ventricular fibrillation, that occur during the early hours of the infarct and that can be prevented or treated. <u>Many deaths from acute myocardial infarction are preventable.</u> The availability of advanced life support in a community will be a major factor in preventing the tragic, unnecessary loss of life associated with AMI.

The most important symptom of AMI is chest pain, which occurs in 80 to 90 percent of patients with the disorder. The pain is similar to that of angina, but is more intense, lasts longer (30 minutes to several hours), and is unrelieved with nitroglycerin. It is classically described as severe—"heavy," "squeezing," "crushing," or "tight." Often a patient will use a clenched fist to describe the pain. In approximately 25 percent of patients, the pain will radiate to the arms, most often the left arm, and into the fingers; less commonly, the pain will radiate to the neck, jaw, upper back, or epigastrium. Occasionally an AMI is mistaken by the patient for indigestion. Like angina, the pain of AMI is not influenced by coughing, deep breathing, or other body movements. The condition may occur at rest or after a heavy meal. The patient with AMI may have a history of angina; thus, angina may be a warning of a possible future AMI. Table 6.2 illustrates the differences between the pain of angina and the pain of AMI.

TABLE 6.2
Signs and Symptoms of Angina Pectoris and Acute Myocardial Infarction

Presenting Signs and Symptoms	Angina Pectoris	Acute Myocardial Infarction
Pain		
Intensity	Mild to moderate	Very severe, intense
Duration	3 to 5 minutes	30 minutes to several hours
Precipitating factors	Specific, predictable physical or emotional stress	No specific predictable factor
Relieving factors	Rest Nitroglycerin	None
Associated symptoms	May be none	Diaphoresis Nausea and vomiting Fear of impending doom

Approximately 10 to 20 percent of patients with AMI do not experience chest pain. This is commonly known as a "silent" AMI. The incidence of painless AMI rises sharply with age; in the elderly patient, AMI may present instead with sudden shortness of breath progressing to pulmonary edema, sudden loss of consciousness, unexplained drop in blood pressure, apparent stroke, or confusion. Other symptoms commonly associated with AMI are diaphoresis (profuse sweating), dyspnea, nausea, vomiting, extreme weakness or fatigue, dizziness, and palpitations.

The physical findings of AMI may be few and will vary with the site and extent of cardiac muscle damage and the amount of sympathetic nervous system response. Therefore, diagnosis in the field will depend primarily on the history of the current complaint. Treatment and stabilization should be started immediately in any middle-aged patient who complains of chest pain. A detailed history and physical examination should be given second priority.

The patient with AMI usually appears anxious or frightened. If the patient is hypoxic, he or she may also appear confused, irritable, or restless. The skin may be pale, cold, or clammy. Blood pressure may be normal, low (systolic pressure of 90 mm Hg or less) if the cardiac output is below normal, or elevated (greater than 160 mm Hg systolic or 90 mm Hg diastolic) in response to stimulation of the sympathetic nervous system. Likewise, the pulse may be normal, bradycardic (slow) if the parasympathetic nervous system is dominant, or tachycardic (fast) if the sympathetic nervous system is dominant.

Advanced life support (definitive cardiac care) must be initiated immediately on all patients who are suspected of having AMI. It is important for paramedics to remember that more than half the deaths from myocardial infarction occur within the first few hours and that patients often do not call for help until several hours after the pain begins. Early treatment can mean the difference between life and death in an otherwise healthy and relatively young man or woman.

Management of the uncomplicated AMI consists of the following definitive cardiac care procedures. The paramedic should:

- Immediately administer oxygen by mask or nasal cannula. Since oxygen therapy can assist in reducing the incidence of arrhythmias following AMI, it should never be withheld from any patient suspected of the condition. The patient with chronic obstructive pulmonary disease should also receive oxygen. If this patient's respirations become depressed, ventilations can be assisted.
- Initiate an intravenous (IV) line of 5-percent dextrose in water (D5W) using a 250-cubic centimeter (cc) bag and microdrip set. The IV rate should be regulated just enough to keep the vein open, usually between 20 to 30 microdrops per minute.
- Attach monitoring electrodes. Transmit the rhythm strip to the hospital for evaluation if biotelemetry is available.
- Monitor vital signs (blood pressure and pulse) every 5 minutes.
- Administer morphine sulfate for pain relief if ordered by the physician.
- Obtain a more detailed history and perform a physical examination after initial stabilization.
- Transport the patient in a comfortable position, usually semisitting.

Following AMI, the patient's clinical course can take several directions. After hospitalization, the patient's course may remain uncomplicated and the infarcted area may heal. During the first few hours of AMI, arrhythmias may develop. Approximately 70 percent of patients with AMI will develop a ventricular arrhythmia. If a large area of cardiac muscle is infarcted, the pumping ability of the heart can be severely impaired and congestive heart failure will ensue. If more than 40 percent of the left ventricle is lost due to infarction, cardiogenic shock will occur.

Congestive Heart Failure

Heart failure following AMI can be understood as mechanical pump failure, or the inability of the heart to maintain cardiac output adequate to meet the metabolic demands of the body. Congestive heart failure indicates circulatory overload either in the systemic circulation, or in the pulmonary circulation, due to an ineffective pump. As a result there are two types of heart failure: left heart failure (acute pulmonary edema) and right heart failure (chronic congestive heart failure).

In AMI, the primary insult is to the left ventricle, affecting the ability of the ventricle to pump blood effectively. Since the heart is a two-pump system, if the pumping ability of the right ventricle is not compromised as a result of the AMI, a temporary imbalance in the cardiac outputs from both ventricles results. The right heart continues to pump blood as usual; however, the left ventricle is unable to completely eject the blood delivered to it into the systemic circulation. As a result, blood begins to back up behind the left ventricle causing an increase in the pressure in the left atrium and pulmonary vessels; this allows blood to accumulate in the lungs. As the pulmonary blood vessels become increasingly engorged with blood, serum is forced out of the capillaries into the alveolar spaces. The serum mixes with air in the alveolar spaces to produce a foam (pulmonary edema). Because the alveoli are partly filled with fluid, the amount of lung tissue available for gas exchange is greatly reduced, and oxygenation is impaired.

In the early stages of pulmonary edema, the patient may appear restless due to the hypoxia that results from impaired oxygenation. As left heart failure progresses, wheezes and an S3 are present. The patient experiences increasing difficulty in breathing and must literally sit up to breathe (orthopnea). To compensate for the increasing hypoxia, the cardiovascular centers in the brain stimulate the sympathetic nervous system, which produces tachycardia, tachypnea, and increased peripheral vascular resistance. If these compensatory mechanisms fail, hypotension occurs, rales develop, and the patient develops a productive cough of blood-tinged frothy sputum. As the accumulation of pulmonary fluid progresses, hypoxemia may become so severe that the patient becomes cyanotic and the state of consciousness decreases. Patients may be literally drowning in their own secretions. This situation is life threatening and demands immediate emergency intervention.

Treatment of left heart failure (pulmonary edema) is aimed at improving oxygenation, increasing myocardial contractility, and reducing venous return. Management of left heart failure consists of the following definitive procedures. The paramedic should:

- Sit the patient up with the feet dangling. This position is the most comfortable for the patient and is advantageous because it decreases venous return to the heart. The actual work of breathing is thus decreased.
- Administer high-flow oxygen by mask. Occasionally acute pulmonary edema is so severe that respiratory failure occurs. If this happens, intubation and

mechanical ventilation are necessary. Positive pressure ventilation via an oxygen-breathing device such as an Elder valve increases the alveolar pressure and diameter. Alveolar collapse is then reduced and ventilation is improved. In addition, venous return is decreased as a result of the increase in intrathoracic pressure.
- Initiate an IV with D5W to keep open.
- Apply monitoring electrodes. Because hypoxia and metabolic acidosis accompany acute pulmonary edema, these patients are predisposed to arrhythmias.

The following drugs may be ordered:

- Morphine sulfate. Morphine is a mainstay in the management of acute pulmonary edema because of its vasodilation, analgesic, and sedative effects. It is recommended that initially a small dose of 4 to 5 milligrams (mg) be given IV. If substantial improvement has not occurred and hypotension has also not occurred, morphine can be repeated in increments until the symptoms of acute respiratory distress are relieved.
- Aminophylline. Aminophylline can be beneficial in the treatment of acute pulmonary edema by causing bronchodilation and increasing cardiac output. Add 200 to 500 mg of aminophylline to 100-cc D5W and infuse at a rate of 20 mg/minute.
- Furosemide (Lasix). Furosemide is a potent, rapid-acting diuretic given IV to decrease intravascular volume. Action begins within 5 to 15 minutes following the injection. Dosage ranges from 20 to 80 mg IV push.
- Digoxin. Digoxin is used in acute pulmonary edema as an adjunct to oxygen, morphine, and furosemide. Digoxin serves to increase contractility of the heart. Where prolonged transport is necessary, digoxin 0.5 to 0.75 mg may be given slowly IV.

Rotating tourniquets can also be employed using the following guidelines:

- Apply tourniquets to three of the four extremities as proximal to the torso as possible.
- Apply tourniquets tightly enough to obstruct venous return but not arterial blood flow.
- Check for presence of distal pulses after each tourniquet is applied.
- Every 10 to 15 minutes, remove a tourniquet from one extremity and secure it to a free extremity. The IV arm may be used if a superficial vein, such as a hand vein, has not been used.
- Rotate the tourniquets in a clockwise direction.

The paramedic should then transport the patient. Monitor vital signs every 5 minutes.

Usually, right heart failure follows left heart failure. As blood backs up from the heart into the lungs, the right side of the heart must work harder to pump blood into the already engorged pulmonary vessels. Eventually the right heart can no longer keep up with the increased workload and fails. When right heart failure occurs, blood backs up behind the right ventricle and increases the pressure in both the right atrium and the systemic veins.

As a direct result of right heart failure, venous return is impeded, and organs become congested. This is manifested by distended jugular veins and the development of body edema. The increased venous pressure forces serum through the capillary walls into the subcutaneous tissues, producing pitting edema. (The existence of this type of edema is confirmed by the pit that forms when pressure is applied.) In ambulatory patients, edema usually first occurs in the dependent parts of the body—the hands and feet—then over the entire body (anasarca). Edema may also be present in the presacral region in recumbent patients.

Increased pressure in the hepatic veins results in liver engorgement, causing the liver to become enlarged and tender. As venous congestion becomes severe, serum may be forced into the abdomen (ascites), pleural cavity (pleural effusion), and pericardial cavity (pericardial effusion).

The development of right heart failure can actually improve left heart failure. Because the right heart is unable to pump blood to the lungs efficiently, pulmonary congestion may actually decrease—thus improving the symptoms of dyspnea of heart failure.

Treatment and management of the patient in congestive heart failure are aimed at decreasing intravascular volume and correcting hypoxia. The paramedic should, first, sit the patient up and administer oxygen. The patient's heart rate should be monitored, as monitoring is indicated in any patient with significant cardiac disease. If signs of left heart failure are present, the patient should be treated as in pulmonary edema (see Table 6.3).

TABLE 6.3
Treatment of Acute Pulmonary Edema

Therapeutic Goal	Therapy	Principle	Precaution
Improvement in oxygenation	Patient sits up	Decreases work of breathing and venous insert	Use position cautiously if hypotension is present
	High flow oxygen	Reverse hypoxemia and prevent metabolic acidosis	Oxygen mask may be frightening to "suffocating" patient
	Positive-pressure ventilation	Decreases fluid and collapse; decrease venous return	

Therapeutic Goal	Therapy	Principle	Precaution
	Aminophylline	Bronchodilator	Will cause hypotension and ventricular arrhythmias if given too rapidly
Reduction of venous return	Morphine sulfate	Causes vasodilation and reduces venous return; decreases anxiety	May cause hypotension and respiratory depression; monitor vital signs
	Furosemide	Rapid diuresis	If given in excessive amounts, can result in hypotension and electrolyte depletion; monitor vital signs
	Rotating tourniquets	Causes venous pooling in extremities	May be uncomfortable; when using tourniquets, remove one at a time at 15-minute intervals to avoid overloading pulmonary circulation again
Increase in myocardial contractility	Digoxin	Increases force of contraction	Monitor for arrhythmias

Cardiogenic Shock

When the heart is damaged so badly that it can no longer pump enough blood to maintain adequate tissue perfusion, cardiogenic shock occurs. Cardiogenic shock indicates extensive damage to the myocardium and has a mortality rate of approximately 85 percent.

The signs and symptoms of cardiogenic shock are the same as those found in other types of shock. The clinical picture is characterized by (1) signs of inadequate tissue perfusion such as pallor; cool, clammy skin; mental confusion; restlessness; and cyanosis of varying degrees and (2) a systolic blood pressure of less than 80 nun Hg. A note of caution: Patients with preexisting hypertension may be in shock although their systolic blood pressure may be higher than 80 mm Hg.

Treatment of cardiogenic shock is aimed at improving peripheral tissue perfusion and increasing myocardial contractility without increasing cardiac work (see Table 6.4). Management of cardiogenic shock consists of the following definitive procedures. The paramedic should:

- Place the patient supine. The Trendelenburg position is not recommended for treating cardiogenic shock.
- Administer high-flow oxygen by mask. Endotracheal intubation may be necessary if the patient becomes unresponsive.
- Start an IV with D5W to keep the vein open.
- Administer the following drugs, if ordered by the physician:

    -- Sodium bicarbonate. Sodium bicarbonate may be ordered to combat metabolic acidosis caused by poor tissue oxygenation.
    -- Norepinephrine (Levophed). Norepinephrine is an alpha stimulator and may be ordered to increase arterial blood pressure. Add 2 mg norepinephrine to 250 cc D5W and infuse IV piggyback via a microdrop administration set at a rate of 30 to 60 microdrops per minute—2 to 4 micrograms (µg) per minute. Titrate flow to the blood pressure response. Norepinephrine must be administered in a large vein because tissue necrosis will occur if the IV infiltrates.
    -- Dopamine (Intropin). Dopamine is a vasopressor that stimulates both alpha and beta receptors. Dopamine increases myocardial contractility and, thus, cardiac output. Dopamine also produces mild vasoconstriction to increase arterial blood pressure. Dopamine has the additional action of dilating the mesenteric and renal vessels to increase blood flow and diuresis. Add 1 ampule (200 mg) of dopamine to 250 cc D5W (3 µg/cc) and infuse at 2 to 5 µg per kilogram (kg) per minute. Titrate the rate to the blood pressure response.
    -- Methylprednisolone (Solu-Medrol). Although the effectiveness of methylprednisolone in cardiogenic shock is unproven, a dose of 30 mg/kg may be given slowly IV push.

Syncope

Syncope, or fainting, is a sudden, temporary loss of consciousness caused by inadequate cerebral blood flow. Although syncope may result from different underlying problems, the most significant causes are cardiac related.

Simple syncope, or vasovagal syncope, is the most common type of syncope and can occur in healthy individuals. Syncope usually follows some emotional stress, such as pain, fright, or the sight of blood. This stress produces reflex peripheral vasodilation and, consequently, pooling of blood in the extremities.

TABLE 6.4
Treatment of Cardiogenic Shock

Therapeutic Goal	Therapy	Principle	Precaution
Correct hypoxia	High flow oxygen Endotracheal intubation		
Correct acidosis	Sodium bicarbonate	To correct lactic acidosis produced by inadequate tissue perfusion	Do not produce sodium overload
Improve circulation	Norepinephrine	Alpha stimulation; increases peripheral vascular resistance; cardiac output remains unchanged	Monitor blood pressure frequently; blood pressure usually raised to 90 mm Hg systolic
			Observe site of administration carefully; infiltration will cause local tissue necrosis
	Dopamine	Alpha-stimulator produces vasoconstriction to increase blood pressure. Beta-stimulator increases cardiac-contractility, increases cardiac output	Monitor blood pressure frequently and titrate to blood pressure response; may produce ventricular arrhythmias

Simple syncope usually occurs when the patient is sitting or standing; consciousness rapidly returns when the patient becomes horizontal. However, the patient may faint again if he or she tries to sit or stand too quickly. The simple faint may occur without warning or may be preceded by a brief period of symptoms such as pallor, weakness, cold sweating, nausea, abdominal discomfort, or blurred vision. Preceding the faint, a tachycardia may be present; however, during the faint, the pulse usually slows to 50 or less.

Syncope of cardiac origin can occur in any position. <u>Syncope that occurs when the patient is lying down is almost always of cardiac origin</u> and indicates a transient decrease in cardiac output. The decrease in cardiac output may be due to bradyarrhythmias, tachyarrhythmias, valvular lesions that obstruct blood flow, or heart block.

Postural syncope occurs when the patient sits or stands up from a supine position. The causes of postural syncope include drugs, chronic disease, and prolonged standing in hot weather.

Carotid sinus syncope is also very common. An individual with a sensitive carotid sinus may faint when the carotid sinus is compressed.

The vagus nerve is stimulated, which slows the heart rate and produces hypotension. These effects combine to produce a faint. The syncopal episode can occur in men while they are shaving and can also be precipitated by the constriction of a tight collar. Patients may also faint after other actions that result in vagal discharge such as violent coughing, laughter, or urination. There are often no warning symptoms.

In taking a history from a patient who has experienced a syncopal episode, the paramedic should find answers to the following questions:
- In what position was the patient when fainting occurred?
- Were there any warning symptoms preceding the faint?
- Did some stressful event precede the faint?
- Has the patient ever fainted before and, if so, under what circumstances?
- Does the patient have a history of cardiac disease?
- Does the patient take any medication?

Regardless of the cause of syncopal episode, there are basic management principles that apply to all forms of syncope. The paramedic should:

- Place the patients supine where they have fallen. The supine position increases cerebral blood perfusion. If patients are placed in a sitting position, they may faint again due to decreased cerebral blood flow. If patients regain consciousness, discourage them from sitting up or standing. Patients should be transported supine to the hospital.
- Establish an airway and administer oxygen.
- Loosen any tight clothing.
- Elevate the lower extremities for 10 to 20 seconds to increase venous return.
- Apply monitoring electrodes to determine the presence of an arrhythmia.
- Initiate an IV of 250 cc D5W to keep open.
- Monitor vital signs.

Other Complications of AMI

Other complications of AMI are ventricular aneurysm and cardiac rupture. Ventricular aneurysm may develop as a result of myocardial infarction. A ventricular aneurysm is a thin-walled bulge in the necrotic area in the wall of the left ventricle. When the ventricle contracts, the aneurysm balloons out; some of the blood pumped into the ventricle flows into the balloon and is not entirely ejected. If the aneurysm occupies 25 percent or more of the ventricular wall, the ventricle pumps even less effectively and congestive heart failure results.

Cardiac rupture may also occur in an infarcted area, but fortunately, this complication is relatively uncommon. Cardiac rupture, in a majority of instances, occurs on the third or fourth day after infarction. The left ventricular wall, papillary muscle, or interventricular septum may rupture following AMI. If the left ventricle ruptures, blood escapes into the pericardial sac producing cardiac tamponade. This complication is usually manifested by the acute onset of shock, jugular venous distention, sinus bradycardia, and, ultimately, electromechanical dissociation. Death can occur within 15 minutes unless the tamponade is relieved and the rupture is repaired surgically.

Rupture of the papillary muscle leads to acute mitral insufficiency and produces profound congestive heart failure, shock, and death. Rupture of the interventricular septum results in severe depression of the left ventricle and pulmonary edema that is resistant to therapy. Hypotension and death ultimately result.

Myocardial Trauma

One frequently overlooked complication of blunt chest injury is trauma to the heart and great vessels. Although the heart is fairly resilient, its position behind the sternum makes it vulnerable to blunt impact injuries. Blunt chest trauma most commonly occurs in steering wheel injuries. Myocardial contusions have occurred in automobile collisions at speeds as low as 25 miles per hour. Myocardial injury may even occur with abdominal trauma.

Myocardial injuries tend to be missed because there are often few signs or symptoms of cardiovascular problems on the initial examination. However, the various injuries produced by nonpenetrating injuries can be serious. <u>All patients with major chest wall trauma should be treated as if they have myocardial trauma until it is proven that they do not.</u>

Automobile accidents are the main cause of myocardial trauma. It is important that the paramedic determine how fast the vehicle was moving, with what the vehicle collided, and the direction of impact. Frontal impact injuries are particularly dangerous, because the impact depresses the posterior sternum, which compresses the heart. Major complications of myocardial trauma are myocardial contusion and cardiac tamponade.

Myocardial contusion is often asymptomatic and masked by symptoms of associated injuries. For example, since the cardiac muscle is damaged and necrosis does occur, myocardial contusion can simulate the signs, symptoms, and complications of AMI.

Primary problems associated with myocardial contusion are cardiac arrhythmias and conduction abnormalities. The site of injury influences the type of arrhythmia encountered. Right-sided chest trauma frequently results in atrial arrhythmias and heart block. Left-sided injuries are more likely to result in ventricular fibrillation. Ventricular arrhythmias are treated as if they occurred during AMI (see above); lidocaine is used to control premature ventricular contractions and countershock is used to control ventricular fibrillation.

An accumulation of blood in the pericardial sac is called cardiac tamponade. Tamponade can be caused by severe myocardial contusion or a tear in a great vessel at the point where it leaves the pericardial sac. When blood fills the pericardial sac, the heart is unable to fill completely, and cardiac output is reduced. As a result, atrial pressure falls and venous pressure rises. Jugular neck vein distention is also present. Pulse pressure (the difference between systolic and diastolic pressure) narrows as the stroke volume falls. Shock is frequently far greater than expected from the amount of blood lost. Blood in the pericardial sac muffles the heart sounds, which will sound more distant upon auscultation.

Cardiac tamponade is a dire emergency. Tamponade must be rapidly treated by removing blood from the pericardial sac (pericardiocentesis). This procedure should be performed in the emergency department under controlled conditions. Therefore, a patient suspected of having a cardiac tamponade must be transported immediately to the hospital. If the patient is unconscious and pulseless, the paramedic should begin cardiopulmonary resuscitation.

Hypertensive Emergencies

Approximately 21 million Americans are afflicted with hypertension (high blood pressure). Hypertension is responsible for more than 20,000 deaths in this country annually. In addition, hypertension is a major risk factor for AMI and cerebrovascular accident (stroke).

Hypertension is usually defined as a resting blood pressure in excess of 140/95 nun Hg. Anxiety, emotional stress, pain, and physical exercise can cause a transient elevation of the blood pressure level, but a persistent elevation of the diastolic pressure indicates hypertensive disease. Left untreated, hypertension significantly shortens life span, and leads to other medical problems.

When the arterial blood pressure rises abruptly to a level of greater than 200/130 Hg, and persists for a prolonged period, a hypertensive crisis is said to be present. A hypertensive crisis imminently threatens the integrity of the patient's cerebral and cardiovascular systems. Frequently, but not always, an acute hypertensive crisis is accompanied by severe headache, irritability, nausea, and vomiting. These symptoms are followed by confusion, convulsions, and coma. Acute hypertensive crises may be complicated by acute pulmonary edema or by intracranial hemorrhage. In such cases, it is essential that the blood pressure be reduced promptly under controlled conditions in the hospital. In the field, only supportive measures are feasible. To support the patient in the field, the paramedic should:

- Secure an airway and administer oxygen
- Initiate an IV with D5W to keep open
- Apply monitoring electrodes
- Monitor vital signs every 5 minutes
- Transport the patient to the hospital

UNIT 4 – READING AND UNDERSTANDING A NORMAL EKG

Fundamental information on reading and understanding an EKG is discussed in this unit, including electrophysiology, components of the EKG record, and interpreting the EKG strip.

Electrophysiology

Each living cell of the body that has the capacity to react to a stimulus is said to be resting or polarized. The inside of the resting cell is electronegative in comparison to the outside of the cell, which is electropositive. This difference can be attributed to the intracellular and extracellular concentration of electrolytes. The semipermeable cell membrane is the main regulator of the resting or polarized state.

When a cell is stimulated to contract, the depolarization process begins. The cell membrane becomes more permeable to extracellular electrolytes, and a shift in electrical charges occurs. The inside of the cell thus becomes electropositive and the outside, electronegative. The wave of depolarization moves across the cell causing the cell to contract. After contraction, a negatively charged wave spreads through the fiber and returns the cell to its original electronegative state. The return of the cell to its resting state is called repolarization. The cell is again polarized and may be stimulated again.

All cells of the body—except cardiac cells—require a stimulus to depolarize. The specialized cardiac cells possess the property of automaticity—that is, they can spontaneously depolarize or contract. If the depolarization of one cell is strong enough, it can influence the contraction of the adjacent cells. Why, then, does the heart beat rhythmically instead of chaotically? The answer is that not all cardiac cells depolarize or contract at the same time.

Normally, the cells of the SA node depolarize faster than any other cells of the heart—at a rate of 60 to 100 times per minute. The SA nodal cells stimulate the other cells of the conduction system in an organized manner. Thus, because the SA nodal cells depolarize faster, the SA node becomes the pacemaker of the heart.

From the SA node, the depolarization wave spreads through the atria and causes them to contract. The atrial muscles are not connected to the ventricular muscles, therefore, the contraction of the atrial muscles will not stimulate the ventricular muscles to contract. There are three atrial internodal pathways leading from the SA node that carry the electrical impulse to the AV node.

From the AV node, the impulse travels to the bundle of His. From the bundle of His, the impulse is conducted to the right and left bundle branches, which, in turn, conduct the impulse to the Purkinje fibers. Stimulation of the Purkinje fibers results in ventricular contraction.

If the SA node starts to depolarize more slowly than any of the other cells, it will no longer be the pacemaker. At that time secondary pacemakers take over—such as the AV node or the bundle branches. The AV node depolarizes 40 to 60 times per minute, and the bundle branches depolarize at a rate of 20 to 40 times per minute. Ischemia, hypoxia, acidosis, or electrolyte imbalances can stimulate the ventricular and atrial cells to act as pacemakers and depolarize spontaneously. A pacemaker that occurs outside the normal conduction pathway is identified as an ectopic focus.

Atrial and ventricular depolarization are electrical events that can be sensed by electrodes on the skin surface. If the electrical impulses are amplified, they can be recorded on the EKG. Therefore, the EKG represents the sum of the electrical activity of the heart, but not of the mechanical activity. The EKG does not reveal how well the heart is contracting.

Components of the EKG Record

During a normal cardiac cycle, the SA node depolarizes first and transmits an electrical impulse to stimulate both atria. This produces a deflection called a P wave. The P wave represents atrial depolarization.

The electrical impulse then reaches the AV node where there is a delay that allows the ventricles to fill with blood. After the pause, the electrical impulse is then conducted to the bundle of His. From the bundle of His, the impulse travels through the right and left bundle branches to the Purkinje fibers and ultimately to the ventricular muscle cells. This process produces the QRS complex that represents ventricular depolarization. It takes approximately 0.10 second for the electrical impulse to depolarize the ventricles. Therefore, the normal time duration for a QRS complex is 0.10 second or less.

After the QRS complex, there is a pause called the S-T segment, which is followed by a T wave. The T wave represents ventricular repolarization. Ventricular repolarization is strictly an electrical event; there is no associated mechanical activity.

Segments and intervals are also identified on the EKG. A segment represents a section of the EKG between waves. The S-T segment represents the time between ventricular depolarization (end of S wave) and ventricular repolarization (beginning of the T wave). An interval is a section of the EKG that includes waves. The P-R interval represents the time duration from atrial depolarization (beginning of the P wave) to the beginning of ventricular depolarization (beginning of the QRS complex). The normal P-R interval duration is 0.12 to 0.20 second. The R-R interval represents the time period between two cardiac cycles (beginning of one QRS complex to the beginning of the subsequent QRS complex).

Reading an EKG Rhythm Strip

An EKG is recorded on graph paper composed of fine vertical and horizontal lines spaced 1 nun apart forming 1 mm squares. At every 5-mm interval, there is a heavy black line. The height or depth of EKG waves may be measured vertically in millimeters and represents a measure of voltage.

The time duration of any wave is measured horizontally. At a normal recording speed of 25 mm/second, each small millimeter square equals 0.04 second. Each large 5-mm square between the heavy black lines equals 0.2 second.

Five basic questions should be answered when an EKG rhythm strip is analyzed systematically:

- What is the rate?
- Is the rhythm regular or irregular?
- Are there P waves and do they have any relationship to the QRS complex?
- What is the P-R interval and is it consistent?
- What is the QRS duration?

<u>What is the rate?</u> The heart rate is the number of cardiac cycles that occur per minute. Both the number of ventricular complexes and the number of P waves that occur per minute should be calculated. Normally, the atrial rate is the same as the ventricular rate.

A normal heart rate is between 60 and 100 beats per minute. A heart rate above 100 beats per minute is identified as a tachycardia. A heart rate below 60 beats per minute is called a bradycardia.

There are several methods that can be used to determine heart rate. Calculator rulers are special devices that can be used to determine rate. However, if a calculator is unavailable during an emergency situation, other methods for calculating heart rates must be used.

At the top of the EKG paper, there are small vertical marks that occur at 3-second intervals. Two of these intervals represent 6 seconds. Ten of the 6-second strips equal 1 minute. To calculate the heart rate, the paramedic should count the number of R-R intervals in the 6-second strip and multiply by 10. This is an "approximate" heart rate and is slower than the actual heart rate. The 6-second count can be used for regular and irregular rhythms.

A third method to calculate heart rate is the triplicate method. The paramedic can find an R wave that falls on a heavy black tine. The next heavy black line is designated as 300 followed by lines designated as 150 and 100. The next three lines after 300, 150, and 100 are designated 75, 60, and 50. Wherever the second R wave falls is the heart rate.

The triplicate method can be used only if the rhythm is regular. If the rhythm is irregular or the heart rate is below 50, the 6-second count must be used.

<u>Is the rhythm regular or irregular?</u> Are the distances between successive R-R intervals equal or unequal? If the R-R intervals are equal, the rhythm is said to be regular. If the duration of the R-R intervals constantly varies, the rhythm is termed irregular.

<u>Are there P waves?</u> The P wave represents atrial depolarization. Therefore, P waves are present on the normal EKG. If P waves are present, are the P-P intervals regular or irregular? Are the P waves consistent in configuration? What is the P:QRS ratio? Is there one P wave for each QRS and does the QRS follow the P wave?

<u>What is the duration of the P-R interval?</u> The P-R interval represents the time from the beginning of atrial depolarization to the beginning of ventricular activation. The normal P-R interval is 0.12 to 0.20 second (3 to 5 little boxes). The P-R interval must be measured to determine if it is prolonged or greater than 0.20 second or if it is shorter than 0.12 second. Two or three successive P-R intervals should be measured to determine if the P-R interval remains constant.

<u>What is the QRS duration?</u> The QRS complex represents ventricular depolarization. The duration of a normal QRS complex is 0.10 second or less (2 1/2 little boxes) and indicates that the impulse has been conducted normally from the AV junction, through the bundle of His, the left and right bundles, and the Purkinje system. A QRS duration of greater than 0.10 second signifies an abnormality in ventricular conduction.

UNIT 5 – ARRHYTHMIA RECOGNITION

Ninety percent of patients with AMI will experience a cardiac arrhythmia sometime during the course of their illness. Fifty percent of the arrhythmias during AMI are life threatening and most frequently occur within the first hours after the infarction. Left untreated, these arrhythmias will lead to cardiac arrest. The cause of death in most AMI patients who die before reaching a hospital is a potentially treatable cardiac arrhythmia.

General Concepts

Arrhythmias are disturbances in rate, rhythm, or conduction; they have many causes. Arrhythmias that occur during AMI are caused usually by either hypoxia in the infarcted muscle or by ischemia in the conducting system.

In addition to necrosis of the heart muscle or ischemia in the conduction system, many other disorders can cause arrhythmias. Imbalances in the autonomic nervous system may result in arrhythmias. Increased sympathetic tone increases the firing rates of both the SA node and secondary pacemakers. In contrast, increased parasympathetic tone decreases the SA node firing rate. However, secondary pacemakers are less sensitive to parasympathetic stimulation. Therefore, when the SA node is excessively slowed by parasympathetic activity, a secondary pacemaker may actually have a faster firing rate and may take over as the pacemaker.

Myocardial stretch may also cause arrhythmias. This most often occurs in the atria as a result of congestive heart failure. In congestive heart failure, the atria distend to accommodate ineffective ventricular pumping.

Hypoxemia (low blood oxygen) and hypercarbia (elevated blood carbon dioxide) can cause arrhythmias as a result of pulmonary edema due to left heart failure and primary lung diseases. Changes in blood pH such as metabolic acidosis and alkalosis also may produce cardiac arrhythmias. When lactic acid accumulates because tissues are poorly oxygenated, metabolic acidosis occurs. Metabolic alkalosis results from excessive antacid ingestion, vomiting, or excessive IV administration of sodium bicarbonate.

Toxic substances released from damaged cells may also affect the electrical conduction system and produce arrhythmias. These products include excessive amounts of potassium, magnesium, lactic acid, adenosine (a nucleic acid component), amino acids, and enzymes. Overdoses of cardiac drugs can likewise produce arrhythmias. These drugs include digitalis, procainamide, quinidine, atropine, lidocaine, epinephrine, dopamine, and isoproterenol.

Serum potassium and calcium imbalances may also cause cardiac arrhythmias. Hyperkalemia, or increased serum potassium, decreases the rate of ventricular depolarization and increases the rate of ventricular repolarization, which widens the QRS complex and produces tall, peaked T waves on the EKG. Hyperkalemia also slows atrial conduction and may cause prolongation of the P-R interval or may cause the P wave to disappear.

Hypokalemia, or low serum potassium, impairs myocardial contractility and increases the durations for depolarization and repolarization. Hypokalemia slows conduction in ventricular muscle. This lengthens and flattens the T wave and produces a

U wave, which is a small positive wave following the T wave. Hypokalemia enhances autoniaticity and leads to increased activity in ectopic pacemakers and produces supraventricular or ventricular arrhythmias.

Serum calcium is important for cardiac excitability and contractility. Hypercalcemia decreases conduction velocity, that is, the QRS duration may be prolonged. AV block may also develop. Hypocalcemia does not usually cause arrhythmias, but it does decrease cardiac contractility.

Arrhythmias are clinically significant. Very slow heart rates or bradycardias (below 40 to 50 beats per minute) reduce cardiac output and frequently precede electrical instability of the heart. With slowing of the sinus rate, ectopic ventricular pacemakers may fire, producing premature ventricular contractions (PVC's) and ventricular arrhythmias.

Very rapid heart rates or tachycardias (over 120 to 140 per minute) increase the workload of the heart, resulting in myocardial ischemia and damage. Tachycardias are also associated with decreased cardiac output. Ventricular electrical instability, manifested by the presence of ectopic beats, is a serious warning that graver prelethal or lethal arrhythmias may follow.

Introduction to Reading Arrhythmias

To recognize abnormal rhythm patterns, a working knowledge of the characteristics of a normal rhythm pattern is essential. A normal heart rate is one between 60 and 100 beats per minute. In a normal rhythm, the R-R intervals are equal; that is, the rhythm is regular. Occasionally, the R-R intervals may vary in regularity up to 0.04 second; however, this is normal and the rhythm is still considered essentially regular. The normal rhythm has P waves that are smoothly rounded and are positive in a lead II. The P waves are consistent in configuration and each precedes a QRS complex. The P-R interval is between 0.12 and 0.20 second and is constant. The QRS duration is 0.10 second or less. The QRS complexes are consistent in configuration. A rhythm strip that meets the above criteria is identified as a normal sinus rhythm.

Abnormalities may be found in any of the above criteria for analyzing a rhythm strip. The heart rate may be below 60 (bradycardia) or above 100 (tachycardia).

An abnormal rhythm is present when the R-R intervals vary by more than 0.04 second. There are regularly irregular rhythms and irregularly irregular rhythms. In a rhythm that is regularly irregular, there is a consistent repetition of R-R interval lengths. This type of rhythm suggests an ectopic focus is firing. In irregularly irregular rhythms, there is no pattern to the R-R interval lengths. An irregularly irregular rhythm suggests atrial fibrillation.

The P wave represents atrial depolarization. When analyzing a rhythm strip, the paramedic must determine if (1) P waves are present, (2) the P waves are similar in size and shape, and (3) there is any relationship between the P waves and the QRS complexes. These determinations will provide information about the pacemaker site and the conduction system. If there are no P waves in the rhythm strip, atrial fibrillation or junctional rhythm may be present. If P waves are negative in lead II, this suggests an ectopic pacemaker in the AV junction. A P wave is abnormal if it is flat or peaked, rather than smoothly rounded, and if it varies in shape and size from cycle to cycle. Distorted, varying P waves indicate several pacemaker sites at different locations throughout the atria (wandering atrial pacemaker). The relationship between the P wave and QRS complex may be altered. If the QRS complex is not preceded by a P wave, the pacemaker site is an ectopic one and not in the SA node. If a P wave is present but not followed by a QRS complex, a block is present somewhere in the AV junction, or below, preventing atrial conduction to the ventricles.

The P-R interval represents the time required for atrial depolarization and conduction of the impulse through the AV junction. The P-R interval is abnormal if it is greater than 0.20 second or less than 0.12 second. When there is disease or damage to the AV node, as sometimes occurs in myocardial infarction, conduction through the junction is slowed even more, and the P-R interval lengthens. A P-R interval greater than 0.20 second is called first-degree AV block and indicates injury to the AV junction. If the P-R interval is less than 0.12 second, this suggests an ectopic pacemaker in the AV junction. If the P-R interval varies from cycle to cycle, this is also abnormal.

The QRS complex represents ventricular depolarization. A normal QRS complex is narrow, has sharply pointed waves, and has a duration of 0.10 second or less. A normal QRS indicates that conduction of the electrical impulse has proceeded normally from the AV junction, through the bundle of His, the left and right bundle branches, and the Purkinje system. An abnormal QRS complex is bizarre in appearance and has a duration longer than 0.10 second. An abnormal QRS complex signifies an abnormality in conduction through the ventricles.

The paramedic should note whether a P wave precedes every QRS complex and whether the P waves and the QRS complexes have a constant relationship or seem to occur independently of one another.

To reiterate, the analysis of every EKG should include the following questions:

- What is the rate?
- Is the rhythm regular or irregular?
- Are there P waves? Is there a P wave before every QRS complex and a QRS complex after every P wave? Based on this, what is the pacemaker site?
- What is the P-R interval?
- Are the QRS complexes normal or abnormal in shape and duration?

In analyzing a rhythm strip, the paramedic must beware of artifacts. A straight line EKG with an alert, communicative patient usually indicates a loose or disconnected electrode—not asystole. Likewise, a wavy baseline simulating ventricular fibrillation may be caused by patient movement or muscle tremor. The paramedic should always observe the patient. A dangerous-looking EKG in an alert patient who is in no obvious distress should indicate to the paramedic that the electrode placement should be rechecked.

System for Identification of Arrhythmias

Rate
    Ventricular
    Atrial

Rhythm
    Ventricular (R-R interval)

Regular

Irregular

Regular irregularity

Irregular irregularity

Atrial
    Regular
    Irregular

Regular irregularity

Irregular irregularity

P Waves
    Configuration
    Relationship to QRS

P-R Interval
    Duration
    Consistency

QRS Complex
    Duration
    Relationship to P wave

GLOSSARY OF HEART TERMS

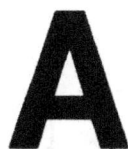

ADRENAL GLANDS *(ah-dre'nal)*
A pair of endocrine (hormone-secreting) glands that sit atop the kidneys. The inner portion of each—the adrenal medulla—secretes norepinephrine and epinephrine. Epinephrine is a heart stimulant and norepinephrine is a powerful blood vessel constrictor. The outer shell—the adrenal cortex—secretes aldosterone, cortisone, and other steroid hormones that influence the body's handling of salt, water, carbohydrates and other aspects of metabolism.

ADRENALIN *(ah-dren'ah-lin)*
See Epinephrine.

ADRENERGIC BLOCKING AGENTS *(ad"ren-er'jik)*
Drugs which block the normal response of an organ or tissue to nerve impulses transmitted by the adrenergic nervous system (more or less the same as the sympathetic nervous system). Blocking adrenergic nerves to the heart and blood vessels tends to decrease heart rate and the vigor of heart contraction and to suppress the constriction of blood vessels. Adrenergic blocking agents are often used to treat angina pectoris (since by reducing heart work they reduce its need for oxygen). Some are also used to treat arrhythmias and to control high blood pressure, especially when it is accompanied by a hyperactive heart.

There are two classes of these drugs, alpha- and beta-adrenergic blocking agents: Both can be used in cardiovascular disorders, although beta-adrenergic blocking agents are used more often; of these, propranolol is the most common.

AGE-ADJUSTED DEATH RATE
See Mortality Rate, Age-Adjusted.

AGE-SPECIFIC DEATH RATE
See Mortality Rate, Age-Specific.

ALDOSTERONE *(al-dos'ter-on OR al"do-ster'on)*
A hormone secreted by the adrenal cortex that promotes the retention of salt and water by the kidneys. Aldosteronism, or excessive secretion of this hormone, may cause an increase in blood pressure. In this case drugs known as aldosterone antagonists can be given; one example is spironolactone.

ALDOSTERONISM *(al"do-ster'on-izm")*
See Aldosterone.

AMINE *(ah-meen' OR am'in)*
An organic compound that may be derived from ammonia by the replacement of one or more of the hydrogen atoms by hydrocarbon fractions.

ANEURYSM *(an'u-rizm)*
A ballooning-out of the wall of a vein, an artery or the heart due to weakening of the wall by disease, traumatic injury or an abnormality present at birth.

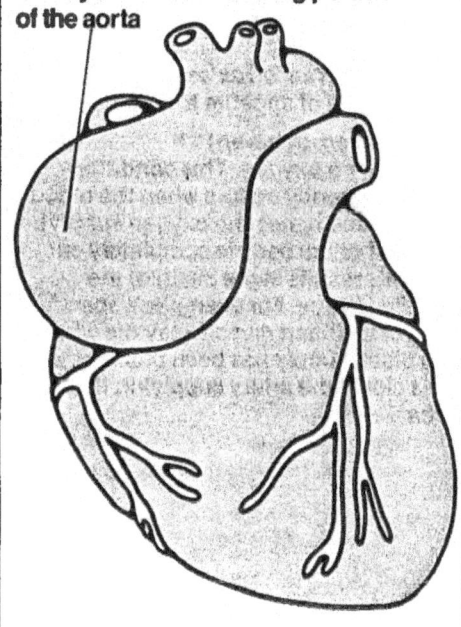

aneurysm of the ascending portion of the aorta

ANGINA PECTORIS *(an-ji'nah OR an'ji-nah pek'tor-is)*
An episode of chest pain due to a temporary discrepancy between the supply and demand of oxygen to the heart. This may be due to low oxygen levels in the blood (from smoking or respiratory disease), to a restricted bloodflow to the heart (coronary insufficiency) or to an increase in heart work beyond normal levels. Most often, angina pectoris is a chronic condition caused by a blood supply restricted by hardening and narrowing of the coronary arteries supplying the heart muscle (coronary atherosclerosis).

An angina attack is not to be confused with a heart attack (myocardial infarction), which results from a severe and prolonged lack of oxygenated blood to a part of the heart.

ANGIOCARDIOGRAPHY *(an"je-o-kar"de-og'rah-fe)*
A diagnostic method involving injection of an x-ray dye into the bloodstream. Chest x-rays taken after the injection show the inside dimensions of the heart and great vessels outlined by the liquid.
See Cineangiography.

ANOREXIA *(an"o-rek'se-ah)*
Lack or loss of appetite for food.

ANOXIA *(an-ok'se-ah)*
Literally, no oxygen. This condition most frequently occurs when the blood supply (and hence the oxygen supply) to a part of the body is completely cut off. This results in the death of the affected tissue. For example, a specific area of the heart muscle may die when the blood supply has been blocked, as by a clot in the artery supplying that area.

ANTIARRHYTHMIC DRUGS *(an"ti-ah-rith'mic)*
Drugs which are used to treat disorders of the heart rate and rhythm. The drugs lidocaine, procaine amide, quinidine, digitalis, and propranolol are often given to correct arrhythmias. Atropine and isoproterenol are used in cases of abnormally slow heart rates.

ANTICOAGULANT *(an"ti-ko-ag'u-lant)*
A drug which delays clotting of the blood (coagulation). When given in cases of a blood vessel plugged up by a clot, it tends to prevent new clots from forming, or the existing clots from enlarging, but does not dissolve an existing clot. Examples are heparin and coumarin derivatives.

ANTIHYPERTENSIVE DRUGS *(an"ti-hi"per-ten'siv)*
Drugs which can be used to control high blood pressure (hypertension). Those most often given are the diuretics (primarily the thiazides), which promote the natural elimination of excess fluids in the tissues and circulation. Some of the other major antihypertensive drugs lower blood pressure by their direct or indirect dilating effect on the arteries. Hydralazine, for example, directly relaxes the tiny muscles in the artery walls. Other drugs block or damper the nerves which signal the arteries to constrict. Some of these are reserpine, methyldopa and guanethidine. The drug propranolol slows the heartbeat, decreases the force of the heart's contraction and thus lowers the blood pressure.

ANXIETY *(ang-zi'e-te)*
A feeling of apprehension.

AORTA *(a-or'tah)*
The main trunk artery which receives blood from the left ventricle of the heart. It originates from the base of the heart, arches up over the heart like a cane handle, and passes down through the chest and abdomen in front of the spine. It gives off many lesser arteries which conduct blood to all parts of the body except the lungs.

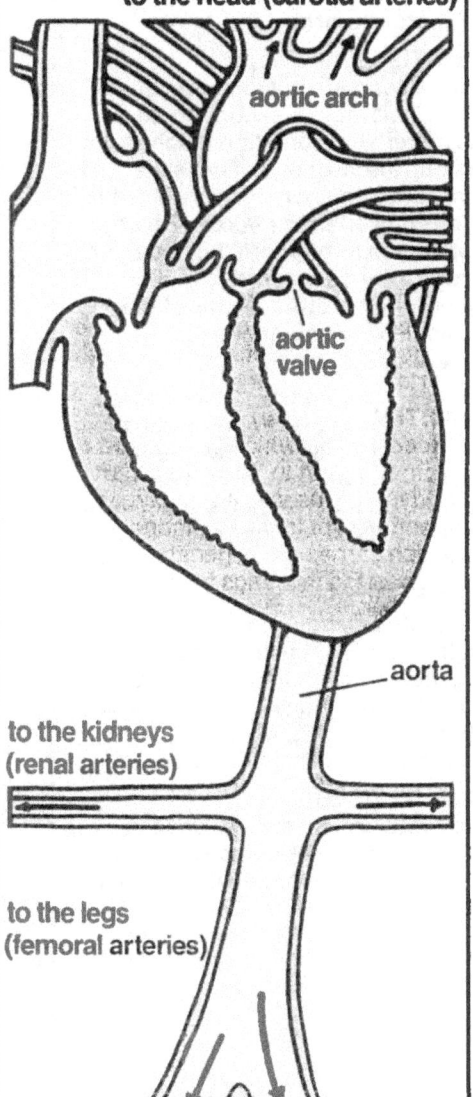

AORTIC ARCH *(a-or'tik)*
The part of the aorta, or large artery leaving the heart, which curves up like the handle of a cane over the top of the heart.

AORTIC INSUFFICIENCY *(a-or'tik in"su-fish'en-se)*
An improper closing of the valve between the aorta and the left ventricle of the heart permitting a backflow of blood.

AORTIC STENOSIS *(a-or'tik stenos'sis)*
A narrowing of the valve opening between the left ventricle of the heart and the large artery called the aorta. The narrowing may occur at the valve itself or slightly above or below the valve. Aortic stenosis may be the result of scar tissue forming after a rheumatic fever infection, or may have other causes.

AORTIC VALVE *(a-or'tik)*
Valve at the junction of the aorta, or large artery, and the left ventricle of the heart. Formed by three opposing cup-shaped membranes, it allows the blood to flow from the heart into the aorta and prevents a backflow. **See Valve.**

AORTOGRAPHY *(a"or-tog'rah-fe)*
X-ray examination of the aorta (main artery conducting blood from the left ventricle of the heart to the body) and its main branches. This is made possible by the injection of a dye which is opaque to x-rays.

APEX *(a'peks)*
The blunt rounded end of the heart, normally directed downward, forward, and to the left.

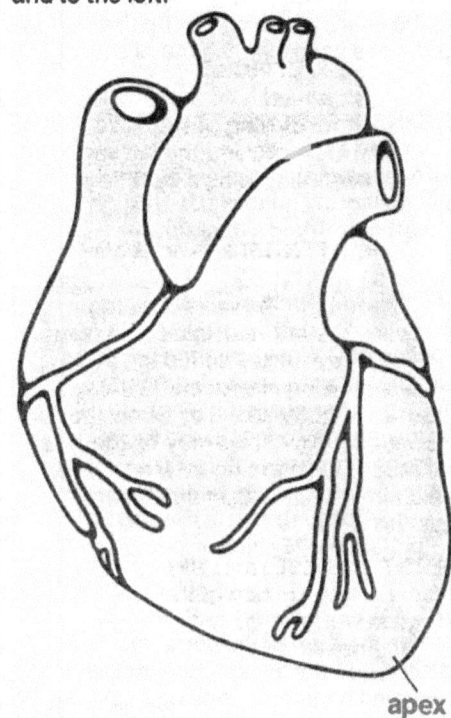
apex

ARCUS *(ar'kus)*
A curved or bowlike structure. **See Corneal Arcus.**

ARRHYTHMIA *(ah-rith'me-ah)*
Any variation from the normal rhythm of the heartbeat.

ARTERIAL BLOOD *(ar-te're-al)*
Oxygenated blood. The blood is oxygenated in the lungs and passes from the lungs to the left side of the heart via the pulmonary veins. It is then pumped by the left side of the heart into the arteries which carry it to all parts of the body. **See Venous Blood.**

ARTERIOLES *(ar-te're-ols)*
The smallest arterial vessels (about 0.2 mm. or 1/125 inch in diameter) resulting from repeated branching of the arteries. They conduct the blood from the arteries to the capillaries.

ARTERIOSCLEROSIS *(ar-te"re-o-skle-ro'sis)*
A group of diseases characterized by thickening and loss of elasticity of artery walls. This may be due to an accumulation of fibrous tissue, fatty substances (lipids) and/or minerals. **See Atherosclerosis.**

ARTERITIS *(ar"te-ri'tis)*
A general term for inflammation of arteries. This may be secondary to some underlying condition (such as an infectious disease) or it may be the primary phenomenon. Primary arteritis includes polyarteritis nodosa (which is disseminated throughout the body), temporal arteritis (occurring at the temples) and aortitis (arteritis of the aorta and its major branches).

ARTERY *(ar'ter-e)*
Blood vessels which carry blood away from the heart to the various parts of the body. They usually carry oxygenated blood except for the pulmonary artery which carries unoxygenated blood from the heart to the lungs for oxygenation. **See Vein.**

ASCHOFF BODIES *(ash'of)*
Spindle-shaped nodules, occurring most frequently in the tissues of the heart, often formed during an attack of rheumatic fever. Named after Ludwig Aschoff (1866-1942), a German pathologist who described them.

ASSIST DEVICES
Special mechanical devices used to provide pumping assistance to a heart weakened by acute heart attack or heart failure.

ASYMMETRIC SEPTAL HYPERTROPHY (ASH) *(a"sim-met'rik sep'tal hi-per'tro-fe)*
Also called idiopathic hypertrophic sub-aortic stenosis (IHSS). A disease of the heart muscle (cardiomyopathy) in which there is an asymmetric enlargement (hypertrophy) of the walls of the left ventricle—the interventricular septum thickens more than the outer wall does. This makes the contraction of the left ventricle less effective and obstructs bloodflow to the aorta (and therefore to all parts of the body including the heart muscle itself). This condition is fairly common, is sometimes hereditary, and can create such symptoms as chest pain and dizziness. Treatment, when necessary, includes surgery, drugs or reduced physical exertion.

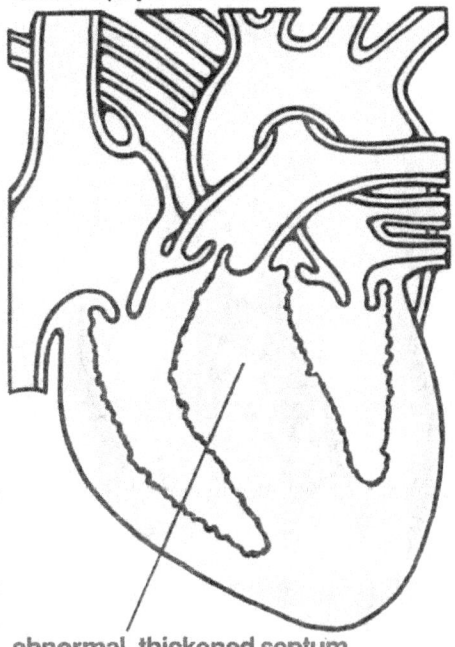

abnormal, thickened septum (asymmetric septal hypertrophy)

ATHEROMA *(ath"er-o'mah)*
Also called plaque. A deposit of fatty (and other) substances in the inner lining of the artery wall, characteristic of atherosclerosis. Plural is **Atheromata** *(ath"er-o-mah'ta)*. See **Atherosclerosis.**

ATHEROSCLEROSIS *(ath"er-o"skle-ro'sis)*
A kind of arteriosclerosis in which the inner layer of the artery wall is made thick and irregular by deposits of a fatty substance. These deposits (called atheromata or plaques) project above the surface of the inner layer of the artery, and thus decrease the diameter of the internal channel of the vessel. See **Arteriosclerosis.**

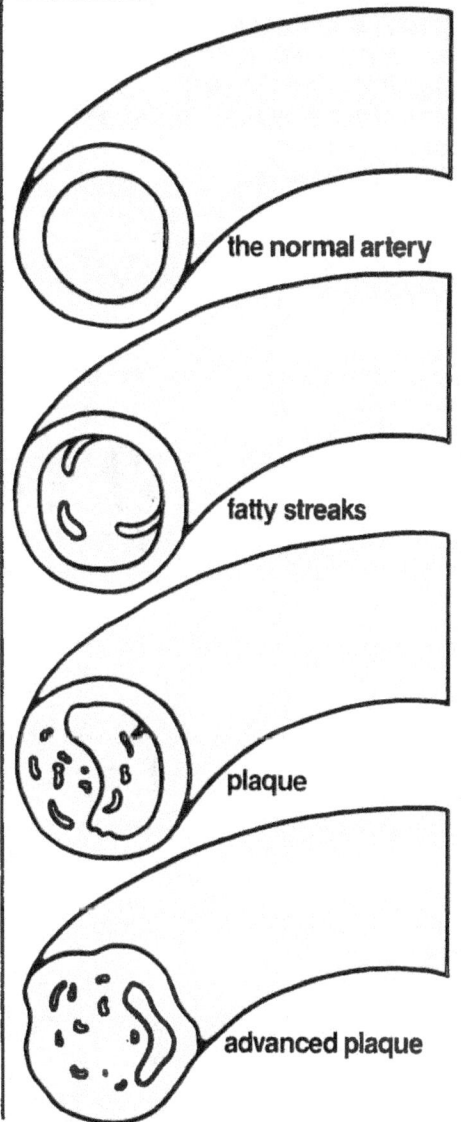

the normal artery

fatty streaks

plaque

advanced plaque

ATRIAL FIBRILLATION (a"tre-al fi-bri-la'shun)
See Fibrillation.

ATRIAL FLUTTER (a'tre-al flut'er)
An arrhythmia which occurs occasionally in healthy hearts, but more commonly in diseased hearts. It results in a rapid regular heartbeat. Drugs are often used to slow the rate.

ATRIAL SEPTUM (a'tre-al sep'tum)
Sometimes called interatrial septum. Muscular wall dividing left and right upper chambers of the heart which are called atria. **See Septum.**

ATRIOVENTRICULAR BUNDLE (a"tre-o-ven-trik'u-lar)
See Bundle of His.

ATRIOVENTRICULAR NODE (a"tre-o-ven-trik'u-lar)
A small mass of special muscular fibers at the base of the wall between the two upper chambers of the heart. It forms the beginning of the Bundle of His which is the only known normal direct muscular connection between the upper and the lower chambers of the heart. The electrical impulses controlling the rhythm of the heart are generated by the pacemaker, conducted through the muscle fibers of the right upper chamber of the heart to the atrioventricular node, and then conducted to the lower chambers of the heart by the Bundle of His. **See Bundle of His and Pacemaker.**

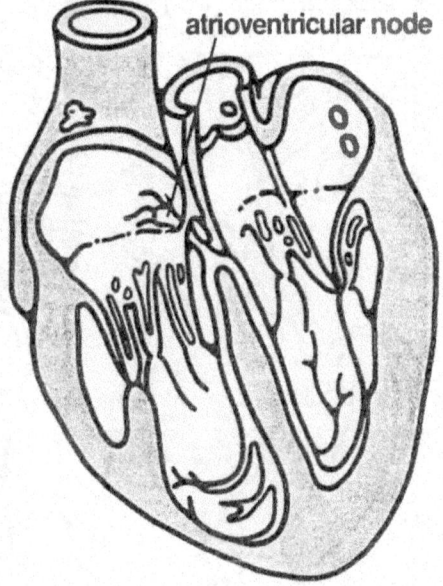

ATRIOVENTRICULAR VALVES (a"tre-o-ven-trik'u-lar)
The two valves, one in each side of the heart, between the upper and lower chambers. The one in the right side of the heart is called the tricuspid valve, and the one in the left side is called the mitral valve. **See illustration inside front cover.**

ATRIUM *(a'tre-um)*
Formerly "auricle." One of the two upper chambers of the heart. The right atrium receives unoxygenated blood from the body. The left atrium receives oxygenated blood from the lungs.

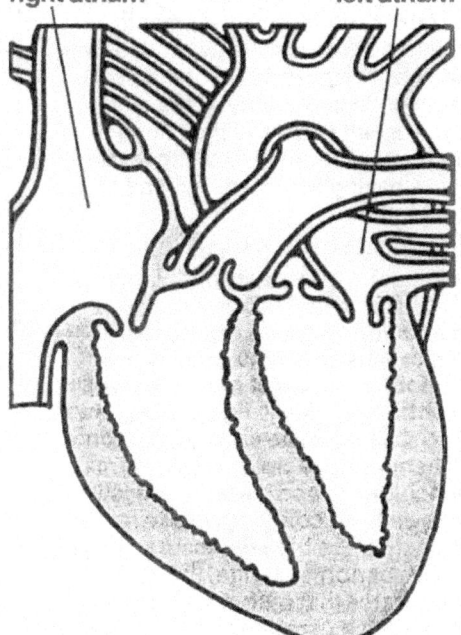

ATROPINE *(at'ro-peen)*
A drug used to treat, among other things, an abnormally slow heart rate; an antiarrhythmic drug.

AUENBRUGGER, LEOPOLD JOSEPH (1722-1809)
Austrian physician who invented the technique of tapping the surface of the body to determine the condition of organs beneath. The technique is called percussion.

AURICLE *(aw're-kl)*
Archaic term for atrium.

AUSCULTATION *(aws"kul-ta'shun)*
The act of listening to sounds within the body, usually with a stethoscope.

AUTONOMIC NERVOUS SYSTEM *(aw"to-nom'ik)*
Sometimes called the involuntary nervous system. The nerves of this system regulate tissues and functions not normally under conscious control (heartbeat, blood pressure, etc.). It consists of two divisions, the sympathetic and parasympathetic, which usually have opposing effects on the cardiovascular system: the sympathetic nerves, when stimulated, tend to increase heart rate, constrict blood vessels, and raise blood pressure; the parasympathetic tend to slow the heart rate, relax blood vessels, and lower blood pressure.

A-V BUNDLE
See Bundle of His.

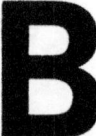

BACTERIAL ENDOCARDITIS *(bak-te're-al en"do-kar-di'tis)*
An inflammation of the inner layer of the heart caused by bacteria; it may be a complication of another infectious disease, an operation or injury. The lining of the heart valves is most frequently affected, most commonly valves with previous damage from rheumatic disease or congenital abnormality.

BARLOW'S SYNDROME *(bar'loz)*
Also called floppy mitral valve syndrome as well as systolic click-murmur syndrome, billowing mitral leaflet syndrome, and prolapsed mitral valve leaflet syndrome (among other terms). A structural alteration of the mitral valve (which normally permits a one-way flow of blood from the left atrium down to the left ventricle of the heart) leading to stretching and weakness of the cusps or valve leaflets. Thus when the heart pumps, some of the blood leaks back into the left atrium instead of being pushed through the aorta to the body.

This syndrome is associated with unusual chest discomfort and arrhythmias.

BARORECEPTORS *(bar"o-re-sep'torz)*
Sensory nerve endings which respond to changes in pressure, as those in the walls of blood vessels.

BEHAVIOR, TYPE A AND TYPE B
Two kinds of behavior patterns, as recognized in medicine. Type A behavior is characterized by high degrees of competitiveness, aggressiveness and feelings of the pressure of time. This type of behavior is thought by some cardiologists to be a risk factor in the development of coronary heart disease. Individuals with the converse Type B behavior are more easygoing and contemplative and more easily satisfied.

BENZOTHIADIAZIDES *(ben"zo-thi"ah-di'ah-sidz)*
See Thiazides.

BETA-BLOCKING AGENTS *(bay'tah)*
Also called beta-adrenergic blocking agents. **See Adrenergic Blocking Agents.**

BICUSPID VALVE *(bi-kus'pid)*
Usually called mitral valve. A valve of two cusps or triangular segments, located between the upper and lower chambers in the left side of the heart. However, in cardiology a "bicuspid valve" usually refers to the common congenital abnormality of the aortic valve's having two cusps instead of its usual three.

BIOFEEDBACK *(bi"o-feed'bak)*
A technique using instrumentation to provide moment-to-moment information about bodily processes which a person is not normally aware of, so that he or she can learn to control them. For example, one setup may include a blood pressure measuring device and colored lights to indicate whether the blood pressure is in the high or normal range. Evidence indicates that biofeedback may be used to teach a person to regulate his or her heart rate, blood pressure, bloodflow, skin temperature, and the activity of the gastrointestinal tract.

This term also refers to the normal and physiologic mechanisms the body uses to regulate myriad physiologic phenomena.

BLOOD PRESSURE
The force the flowing blood exerts against the artery walls. Two pressures are usually measured:
1. The upper, or **systolic**, pressure occurs each time the heart contracts (systole) and pumps blood into the aorta.
2. The lower, or **diastolic**, pressure occurs when the heart relaxes (diastole) and refills with blood flowing in from the large veins, the venae cavae.

The blood pressure is therefore expressed by two numbers, with the upper one over the lower one; for example, 120/80, which is spoken as "120 over 80."

BLUE BABIES
Babies having a blueness of skin (cyanosis) caused by insufficient oxygen in the arterial blood. This often indicates a heart defect, but may have other causes such as premature birth or impaired respiration.

BRADYCARDIA (brad-e-kar'de-ah)
Abnormally slow heart rate. Generally, anything below 60 beats per minute is considered bradycardia.

BRIGHT, RICHARD (1789-1858)
English physician who demonstrated the association of heart disease to kidney disease.

BUERGER'S DISEASE (ber'gerz)
A disease of the blood vessels which is more commonly called thromboangiitis obliterans. **See Thromboangiitis Obliterans.**

BUERGER'S SYMPTOM (ber'gerz)
In thromboangiitis obliterans (Buerger's disease), the pain in the affected leg when the patient is lying down is relieved only by letting the leg hang over the side of the bed. **See Thromboangiitis Obliterans.**

BUNDLE OF HIS (hiss)
Also called atrioventricular bundle or A-V bundle. A bundle of specialized muscle fibers running from a small mass of muscular fibers (atrioventricular node) between the atria of the heart down to the ventricles. It is the only known normal direct muscular connection between the atria and the ventricles, and serves to conduct impulses for the rhythmic heartbeat from the atrioventicular node to the heart muscle. Named after Wilhelm His, German anatomist.

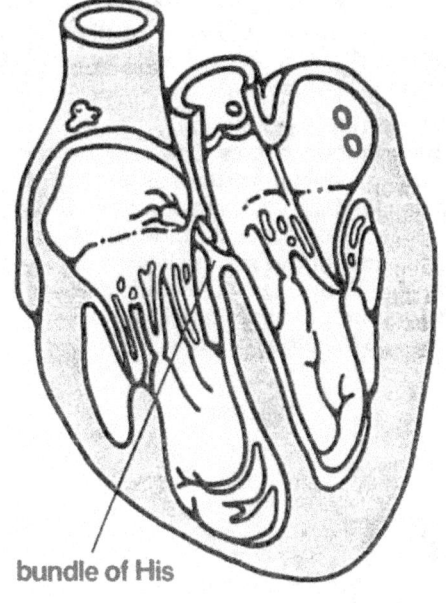

bundle of His

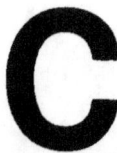

CAESALPINUS, ANDREAS (1519?-1603)
First to use the term "circulation" in connection with the movement of the blood. However, he still believed in many of the classical theories taught by Galen.

CALORIE (kal'o-re)
Sometimes called large or kilocalorie. Unit used to express food energy. The amount of heat required to raise the temperature of 1 kilogram of water 1 degree Centigrade.

A high caloric diet has a prescribed caloric value above the total daily energy requirement. A low caloric diet has a prescribed caloric value below the total energy requirement.

CAPILLARIES (kap'i-lar"ez)
The tiniest blood vessels. Capillary networks connect the arterioles and venules. Capillary walls are composed of a single layer of cells through which oxygen and nutritive materials pass out to the tissues, and carbon dioxide and waste products are admitted from the tissues into the bloodstream.

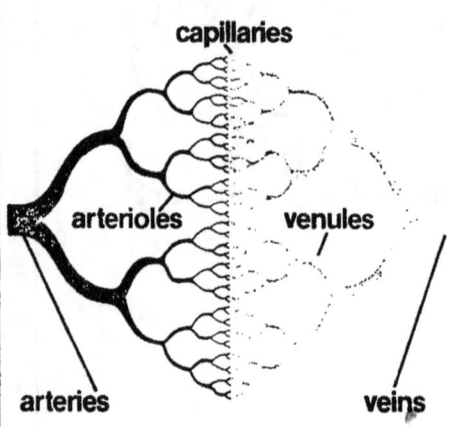

CARBON DIOXIDE (kar'bon di-ox'ide)
A waste product of chemical reactions in the cells. It passes from the cells to the blood which eventually releases it in the lungs to be breathed out.

CARDIAC (kar'de-ak)
Pertaining to the heart. Sometimes refers to a person who has heart disease.

CARDIAC ARREST
Cessation of the heartbeat. As a result, blood pressure drops abruptly and the circulation of the blood ceases. Until recently, this was always fatal. Today, the heart can be stimulated to start beating again and death averted under certain circumstances. **See Cardiopulmonary Resuscitation.**

CARDIAC CYCLE

A cardiac cycle is the series of mechanical and electrical events associated with one heartbeat. One cycle or beat lasts about 0.9 seconds and includes contraction and pumping, relaxation and filling actions.

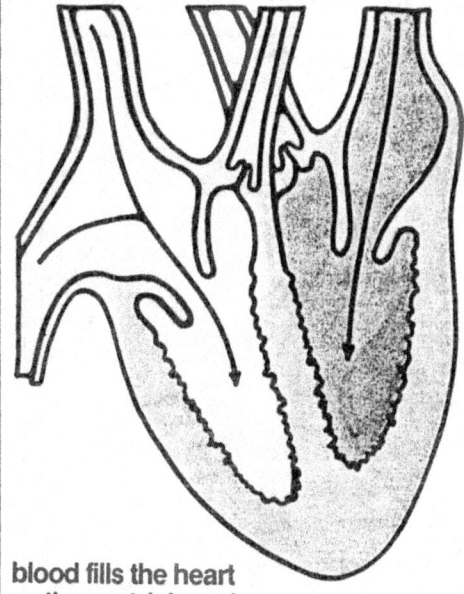

blood fills the heart as the ventricles relax

the ventricles contract and pump the blood out

CARDIAC OUTPUT
The amount of blood pumped by the heart per minute.

CARDIAC RESERVE
The difference between the cardiac output at rest (about 5 quarts pumped by one ventricle per minute) and at the maximum physical effort (as much as 25 quarts per minute or more).

CARDIOLOGIST (kar-de-ol'o-jist)
A specialist in the diagnosis and treatment of heart disease.

CARDIOLOGY (kar"de-ol'o-je)
The study of the heart and its functions in health and disease.

CARDIOMYOPATHY *(kar"de-o-mi-op'ah-the)*
A general diagnostic term for diseases that involve mainly the myocardium (heart muscle) and not other heart structures (such as the valves, coronary vessels or pericardium). They may be caused by known toxic or infectious agents. For the majority of cases, however, the cause is not known.

CARDIOPULMONARY RESUSCITATION (CPR) *(kar"de-o-pul'mo-ner-e re-sus"i-ta'shun)*
Also called Basic Life Support. An emergency measure used by one or two people to artificially maintain another person's breathing and heartbeat in the event these functions suddenly stop. CPR consists of keeping the airway open and performing rescue breathing and external cardiac compression (heart massage) to keep oxygenated blood circulating through the body. **See Heart Massage.**

CARDIOVASCULAR *(kar"de-o-vas'ku-lar)*
Pertaining to the heart and blood vessels.

CARDIOVASCULAR-RENAL DISEASE *(kar"de-o-vas'ku-lar re'nal)*
Disease involving the heart, blood vessels, and kidneys.

CARDIOVERSION *(kar'de-o-ver"zhun)*
The application of very brief discharges of direct-current electricity across the intact chest and into the heart muscle in order to stop a cardiac arrhythmia (rhythm disorder) and allow the normal heart rhythm to take over. This technique is most often used as an emergency measure, but can also be used to correct chronic conditions.

CARDIOVERTER *(kar'de-o-ver"ter)*
An instrument capable of delivering a brief direct-current electric shock. Used to terminate certain cardiac arrhythmias. **See Cardioversion.**

CARDITIS *(kar-di'tis)*
Inflammation of the heart.

CAROTID ARTERIES *(kah-rot'id)*
The left and right common carotid arteries are the principal arteries supplying the head and neck. Each has two main branches, the external carotid artery and the internal carotid artery.

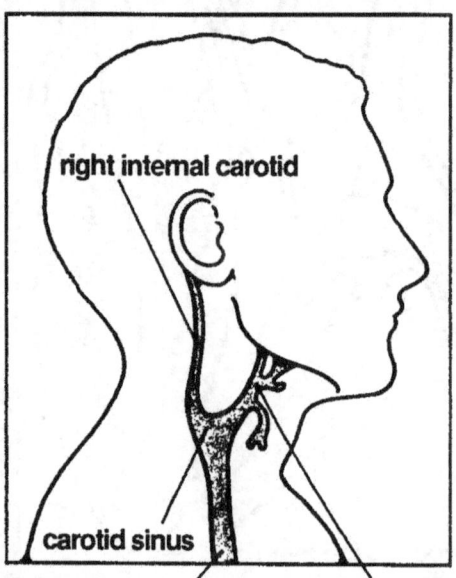

right common carotid artery / right external carotid / right internal carotid / carotid sinus

CAROTID BODY *(kah-rot'id)*
A tiny (5 mm. or 1/5 inch) oval mass of cells located in each carotid sinus, that is, at the branching point in the arteries supplying the head and neck. The carotid bodies contain nerve endings known as chemoreceptors which are sensitive to oxygen and carbon dioxide content and to pH of the blood. For example, when the oxygen content of the blood is reduced, the carotid bodies cause an increase in respiration rate.

CAROTID SINUS *(kah-rot'id si'nus)*
On either side of the neck, a slight dilation at the point where the internal carotid artery branches from the common carotid artery. These arteries supply the head and neck with blood. The carotid sinus contains the carotid body and many baroreceptors, special nerve endings sensitive to changes in blood pressure to keep it relatively constant. For example, if blood pressure starts to rise, baroreceptors in the carotid sinuses are stimulated to reduce the rate and force of heart contraction and to dilate the arteries—thus lowering the blood pressure. **See Carotid Arteries and Carotid Body.**

CATHETER *(kath'e-ter)*
A thin, flexible tube which can be guided into body organs. A cardiac catheter is made of woven plastic, or other material to which blood will not adhere, and is inserted into a vein or artery (usually of an arm or a leg) and gently threaded into the heart. Its progress can be watched on a fluoroscope.

Cardiac catheters can be used for diagnosis (to take samples of blood or pressure readings in the chambers of the heart) or for treatment (to implant the electrodes of a pacemaker or to administer a drug).

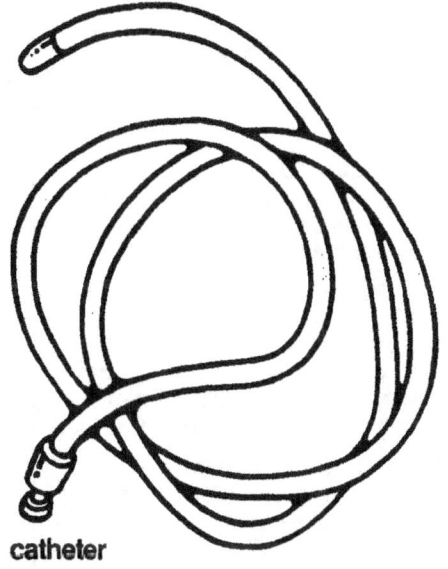

catheter

CATHETERIZATION *(kath"e-ter-i-za'shun)*
In cardiology, the process of introducing a thin, flexible tube (a catheter) into a vein or artery and guiding it into the heart for purposes of examination or treatment.

CEREBRAL VASCULAR ACCIDENT (ser'e-bral OR se-re'bral vas'ku-lar)
Sometimes called cerebrovascular accident, apoplectic stroke, or simply stroke. An impeded blood supply to some part of the brain, generally caused by one of the following four conditions:
1. A blood clot forming in the vessel (cerebral thrombosis).
2. A rupture of the blood vessel wall (cerebral hemorrhage).
3. A piece of clot or other material from another part of the vascular system which flows to the brain and obstructs a cerebral vessel (cerebral embolism).
4. Pressure on a blood vessel as by a tumor.

For illustration see Stroke.

CEREBROVASCULAR (ser"e-bro-vas'ku-lar)
Pertaining to the blood vessels in the brain.

CHAGAS HEART DISEASE (chag'as)
A form of heart disease resulting from an infection by a microscopic parasite found in South America.

CHEMOTHERAPY (ke"mo-ther'ah-pe)
The treatment of disease by administering chemicals. Frequently used in the phrase "chemotherapy of hypertension," i.e., the treatment of high blood pressure by the use of drugs.

CHLOROTHIAZIDE (klo"ro-thi'ah-zid)
One of the thiazide diuretics (drugs which promote the excretion of urine). Sometimes used to treat high blood pressure and edema (waterlogged tissues).

CHOLESTEROL (ko-les'ter-ol)
A fat-like substance found in animal tissue. In blood tests the normal level for Americans is assumed to be between 180 and 230 milligrams per 100 cc. A higher level is often associated with high risk of coronary atherosclerosis.

CHOLESTYRAMINE (ko"les-ti'rah-meen)
A drug used to lower blood levels of the lipid cholesterol. **See Lipid-Lowering Drugs.**

CHORDAE TENDINEAE (kor'di ten'dun-i)
Fibrous chords which serve as guy ropes to hold the valves between the upper and lower chambers. They stretch from the cusps of the valves to muscles called papillary muscles in the walls of the lower heart chambers.

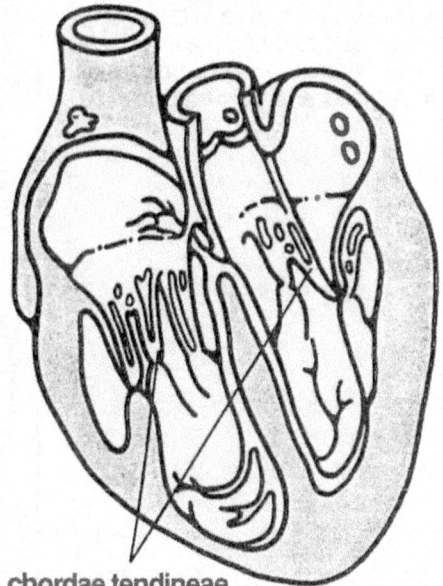

chordae tendineae

CHOREA (ko-re'ah)
Involuntary, irregular twitching of the muscles, sometimes associated with rheumatic fever. Also called St. Vitus Dance, or Sydenham's Chorea.

CINEANGIOCARDIOGRAPHY (sin"e-an"je-o-kar"de-og'rah-fe)
A diagnostic method similar to angiocardiography except that instead of still x-ray pictures, motion pictures of the heart are made by fluoroscopy, as an injected opaque liquid is carried through the heart and blood vessels. **See Angiocardiography.**

CIRCULATORY *(ser'ku-lah-to"re)*
Pertaining to the heart, blood vessels, and the circulation of the blood.

CLAUDICATION *(klaw"di-ka'shun)*
Pain and lameness or limping. Can be caused by defective circulation of the blood in the vessels of the limbs. **See Intermittent Claudication.**

CLOFIBRATE *(klo-fi'brat)*
A drug generally used to lower elevated levels of triglyceride lipids in the blood. **See Lipid-Lowering Drugs.**

CLUBBED FINGERS *(klubd)*
Fingers with a short broad tip and overhanging nail, somewhat resembling a drumstick. This condition is sometimes seen in children born with certain kinds of heart defects and in adults with heart, lung or gastrointestinal diseases. It may also be familial and insignificant.

COAGULATION *(ko-ag"u-la'shun)*
Process of changing from a liquid to a thickened or solid state. The formation of a clot.

COARCTATION OF THE AORTA *(ko"ark-ta'shun of the a-or'ta)*
Literally a pressing together or narrowing of the aorta, the main trunk artery which conducts blood from the heart to the body. One of several types of congenital heart defects.

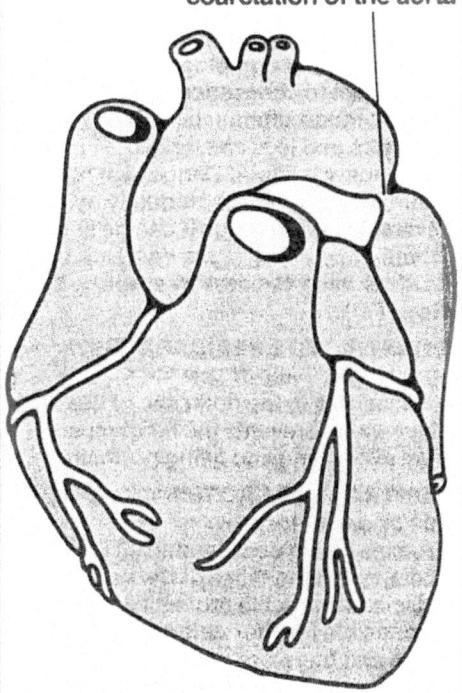

coarctation of the aorta

COLLATERAL CIRCULATION *(ko-lat'er-al ser"ku-la'shun)*
Circulation of the blood through nearby smaller vessels when a main vessel has been blocked up.

COMMISSUROTOMY *(kom"e-shur-ot'o-me)*
An operation to widen the opening in a heart valve which has become narrowed by scar tissue. The individual flaps of the valve are spread apart along the natural lines of their closure by a blunt instrument. This operation was developed to correct rheumatic heart disease. **See Mitral Valvulotomy.**

CONGENITAL ANOMALY *(kon-jen'i-tal ah-nom'ah-le)*
An abnormality present at birth.

CONGESTIVE HEART FAILURE *(kon-jes'tiv)*
"Heart failure" is a condition in which the heart is unable to pump its required amount of blood.

Heart failure is often congestive because loss of pumping power by the heart leads to congestion in the body tissues; fluid accumulates in the abdomen and legs and/or in the lungs (pulmonary edema). Congestive heart failure often develops gradually over several years, although it can be acute (short and severe). It can be treated by drugs or in some cases by surgery. **See Heart Failure.**

CONSTRICTIVE PERICARDITIS *(kon-strik'tiv per"i-kar-di'tis)*
A thickening of the outer sac of the heart which prevents the heart muscle from expanding and filling normally.

CONTRACTILE PROTEINS *(kon-trak'til pro'te-ins)*
Proteins which occur within all muscle fibers, including those of the heart muscle. Contractile proteins are responsible for shortening the muscle fibers and therefore causing the muscle to contract. There are several kinds of contractile proteins.

CORNEAL ARCUS *(kor'ne-al ar'kus)*
A hazy ring around the edge of the cornea (the transparent covering over the front of the eye). It can have a variety of causes, including exposure to irritating chemicals, viral or bacterial infections, and old age. It can also be a normal finding in certain racial backgrounds.

In addition, corneal arcus can be a sign of Type II or Type IV hyperlipoproteinemia, blood-lipid disorders associated with premature development of atherosclerosis (hardening of the arteries).

CORONARY ARTERIES *(kor'o-na-re)*
Arteries, arising from the base of the aorta, which conduct blood to the heart muscle. These arteries, and the network of vessels branching off from them, come down over the top of the heart like a crown (corona).

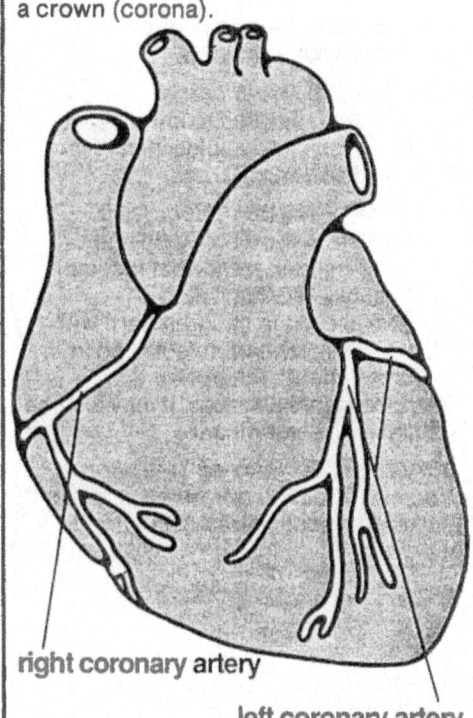

right coronary artery

left coronary artery

CORONARY ARTHEROSCLEROSIS *(ath"er-o"skle-ro'sis)*
Commonly called coronary heart disease. An irregular thickening of the inner layer of the walls of the arteries which conduct blood to the heart muscle. The internal channel of these arteries (the coronaries) becomes narrowed and the blood supply to the heart muscle is reduced. **See Atherosclerosis.**

CORONARY BYPASS SURGERY
(kor'o-na-re bi'pas)
Surgery to improve the blood supply to the heart muscle when narrowed coronary arteries reduce flow of the oxygen-containing blood which is vital to the pumping heart. This reduction in bloodflow causes chest pain and leads to increased risk of heart attack. Thus coronary bypass surgery involves constructing detours through which blood can bypass narrowed portions of coronary arteries to keep the heart muscle supplied. Veins or arteries taken from other parts of the body where they are not essential are grafted onto the heart to construct these detours.

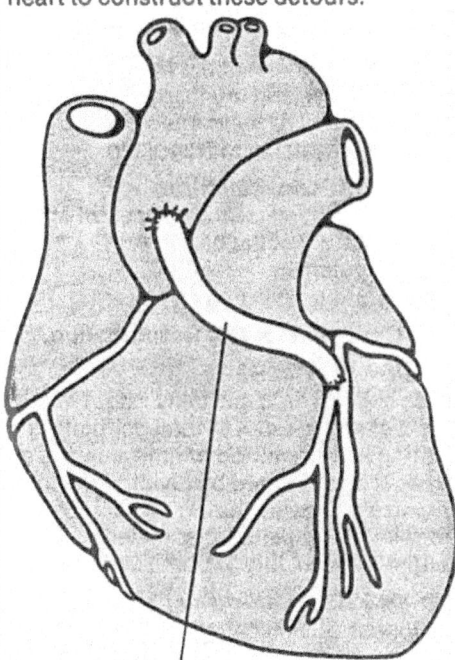

a bypass graft from the aorta to one of the coronary arteries

CORONARY HEART DISEASE
Also called coronary artery disease and ischemic heart disease. Heart ailments caused by narrowing of the coronary arteries and therefore a decreased blood supply to the heart (ischemia).

CORONARY INSUFFICIENCY *(in"su-fish'en-se)*
A condition which occurs whenever the coronary arteries (which supply the heart muscle with blood) do not provide oxygen adequate to the needs of the pumping heart. This may produce chest pain (angina pectoris) or a heart attack, or no pain may occur at all.

"*Acute* coronary insufficiency" is a term used to describe chest pain that is more severe than that of angina pectoris, but in which no heart muscle damage is done (as there would be in a heart attack).

CORONARY OCCLUSION *(o-kloo'zhun)*
An obstruction in a branch of one of the coronary arteries which hinders the flow of blood to some part of the heart muscle. This part of the heart muscle then dies because of lack of oxygen supply. Sometimes called a coronary heart attack or simply a heart attack. **See Heart Attack.**

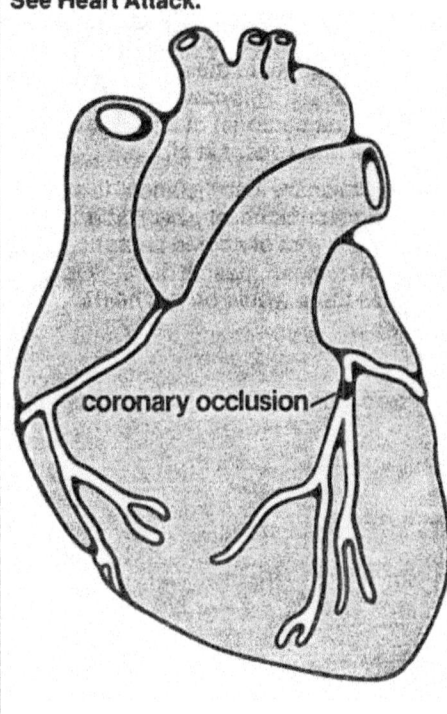
coronary occlusion

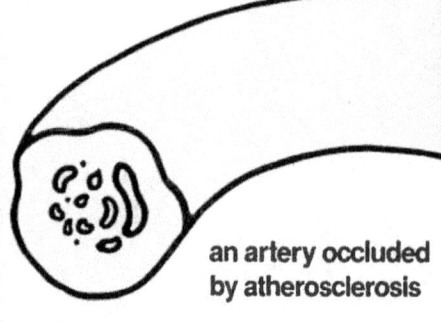
an artery occluded by atherosclerosis

CORONARY THROMBOSIS *(throm-bo'sis)*
Formation of a clot in a branch of one of the arteries which conduct blood to the heart muscle (coronary arteries). A form of coronary occlusion. **See Coronary Occlusion.**

COR PULMONALE *(kor pul-mo-nal'e)*
Heart disease resulting from disease of the lungs or the blood vessels of the lungs. The lung problems cause high blood pressure in the pulmonary vessels (pulmonary hypertension). Thus the right ventricle enlarges because it must work harder to pump blood through the lungs.

CORVISART, JEAN NICOLAS (1755-1821)
One of the earliest of the modern cardiologists, and the first person to call him or herself a "heart specialist." Favorite physician to Napoleon.

COUMARIN *(koo'mah-rin)*
A class of chemical substances which delay clotting of the blood. An anticoagulant.

CPR
See Cardiopulmonary Resuscitation.

CRUDE DEATH RATE
Also called crude mortality rate. The ratio of total deaths to total population during a given period of time, such as a year. It is calculated by dividing the total number of deaths during the year by the mid-year population (estimated population on July 1) of the same year.

CYANOSIS *(si"ah-no'sis)*
Blueness of skin caused by insufficient oxygen in the blood. Oxygen is carried in the blood by hemoglobin, which is bright red when saturated with oxygen. When hemoglobin is not carrying oxygen, it is dark burgundy and is called reduced hemoglobin. The blueness of the skin occurs when the amount of reduced hemoglobin exceeds 5 grams per 100 cc. of blood.

D

DECOMPENSATION *(de"kom-pen-sa'shun)*
Inability of the heart to maintain adequate circulation, usually resulting in a waterlogging of tissues. A person whose heart is failing to maintain normal circulation is said to be "decompensated."

DEFIBRILLATION *(de-fib"ri-la'shun)*
Termination of atrial or ventricular fibrillation. Usually refers to treatment by the application of electric shock (cardioversion). **See Fibrillation and Cardioversion.**

DEPRESSANT *(de-pres'ant)*
Any drug which decreases functional activity.

DESCARTES, RENE (1596-1650)
Author of the first physiology textbook which accepted the theory of the circulation of the blood as described by William Harvey.

DEXTROCARDIA *(deks"tro-kar'de-ah)*
Two different types of congenital phenomena are often described as dextrocardia. The first is a condition more correctly termed "dextroversion" in which the heart is slightly rotated and lies almost entirely in the right (instead of the left) side of the chest. The second is a condition in which the left chambers of the heart are on the right side and the right chambers are on the left side, so that the heart and great vessels present a mirror image of the normal heart.

DIASTOLE *(di-as'to-le)*
In each heartbeat, the period of the relaxation of the heart. Atrial diastole is the period of relaxation of the atria, or upper heart chambers. Ventricular diastole is the period of relaxation of the ventricles, or lower heart chambers. **See Cardiac Cycle.**

DIET *(di'et)*
Daily allowance or intake of food and drink.

DIETETICS *(di-e-tet'iks)*
The science and art dealing with the application of principles of nutrition to the feeding of individuals or groups under different economic or health conditions.

DIETITIAN *(di-e-tish'an)*
One skilled in the scientific use of diet in health and disease.

DIGITALIS *(dij"e-tal'is)*
A drug prepared from leaves of the foxglove plant. Its main effect is cardiotonic, that is, it causes the heart muscle to pump more forcefully and effectively, thereby improving the circulation of the blood and promoting the normal elimination of excess fluid. Digitalis is often used to treat heart failure because it can relieve one of the early effects of the condition—buildup of fluid in the body tissues.

Digitalis is the most frequently used cardiotonic drug; other examples are ouabain and strophanthidin.

DILATION *(di-la'shun)*
A stretching or enlargement of the heart or blood vessels beyond the norm.

DIURESIS *(di"u-re'sis)*
Increased excretion of urine.

DIURETIC *(di"u-ret'ik)*
A medicine which promotes the excretion of urine. These drugs are often used to treat conditions involving excess body fluid such as hypertension and congestive heart failure. One important class of diuretics is the thiazides.

DUCTUS ARTERIOSUS *(duk'tus ar-te"re-o'sis)*
A small duct in the heart of the fetus between the artery leaving the right side of the heart (pulmonary artery) and the artery leaving the left side of the heart (aorta). Normally this duct closes soon after birth. If it does not close, the condition is known as patent or open ductus arteriosus. **See Patent Ductus Arteriosus.**

DYSPNEA *(disp'ne-ah)*
The uncomfortable sensation or awareness of shortness of breath.

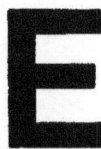

ECG
See Electrocardiogram

ECHOCARDIOGRAPHY *(ek"o-kar"de-og'rah-fe)*
A diagnostic method by which pulses of sound (ultrasound) are transmitted into the body and the echoes returning from the surfaces of the heart and other structures are electronically plotted and recorded. Stop-action or real-time images of the heart can be made into a record of the heart's movements.

ECHOGRAM *(ek'o-gram)*
An image of the heart and great vessels, as would be produced by echocardiography.

ECTOMORPH *(ek'to-morf)*
Wiry body type.

EDEMA *(e-de'mah)*
Swelling due to abnormally large amounts of fluid in the tissues of the body.

EFFORT SYNDROME *(sin'drom)*
A group of symptoms (quick fatigue, rapid heartbeat, sighing breaths, dizziness) that do not result from disease of organs or tissues and that are out of proportion to the amount of exertion required. Often called functional heart disease.

EISENMENGER'S SYNDROME *(i'sen-meng"erz)*
A condition in which there is a large congenital shunting defect complicated by high blood pressure in the vessels of the lungs (pulmonary hypertension). A shunting defect is an abnormal opening between heart chambers (septal defect) or between the great vessels (such as patent ductus arteriosus) such that some oxygen-poor blood gets pumped to the body and some oxygen-rich blood gets pumped to the lungs.

The syndrome is also called Eisenmenger's Reaction. The term **Eisenmenger's Complex** is used only when the defect is in the ventricular septum.

EKG
See Electrocardiogram.

ELECTROCARDIOGRAM *(e-lek"tro-kar'de-o-gram")*
Often referred to as ECG or EKG. A graphic record of the electric currents generated by the heart.

The word "electrocardiogram" most often refers to a resting electrocardiogram, that is, the patient is lying at rest while the recording is being made. The recording can also be made during exercise. **See Exercise Electrocardiogram.**

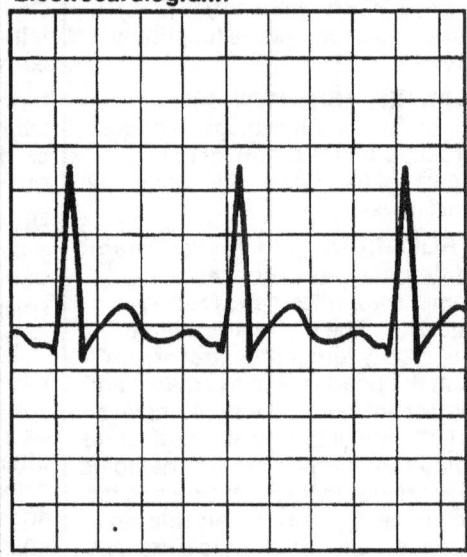

electrocardiogram

ELECTROLYTE *(e-lek'tro-lit)*
A substance which, when dissolved in a liquid, dissociates into ions (positively and negatively charged particles). A solution of electrolytes is capable of conducting an electrical current.

Electrolytes, especially sodium and potassium, occur naturally in the body fluids. Heart disease and medications to treat it can cause abnormal electrolyte concentrations in the body fluids. Physicians sometimes prescribe diet and medications to correct these disordered concentrations.

EMBOLISM *(em'bo-lizm)*
The blocking of a blood vessel by a clot or other substance carried in the bloodstream.

EMBOLUS *(em'bo-lus)*
A blood clot (or other substance such as an air bubble, fat or tumor) which drifts unattached in the bloodstream until it becomes lodged in a small vessel and obstructs circulation. **See Thrombus.**

ENDARTERECTOMY *(end"ar-ter-ek'to-me)*
Surgical removal of the innermost lining (intima) of an artery when it is thickened by fatty deposits (atheroma) and blood clots (thromboses).

ENDOCARDIAL FIBROELASTOSIS *(en"do-kar'de-al fi"bro-e"las-to'sis)*
A heart disease of unknown cause occurring in adults, but mostly in infants. It involves thickening of the lining of the heart chambers (endocardium) with elastic tissue. The thickening is most pronounced in the left ventricle and greatly impairs cardiac function.

ENDOCARDITIS *(en"do-kar-di'tis)*
Inflammation of the inner lining of the heart (endocardium) usually associated with acute rheumatic fever or some infectious agents.

ENDOCARDIUM *(en"do-kar'de-um)*
A thin smooth membrane forming the inner surface of the heart.

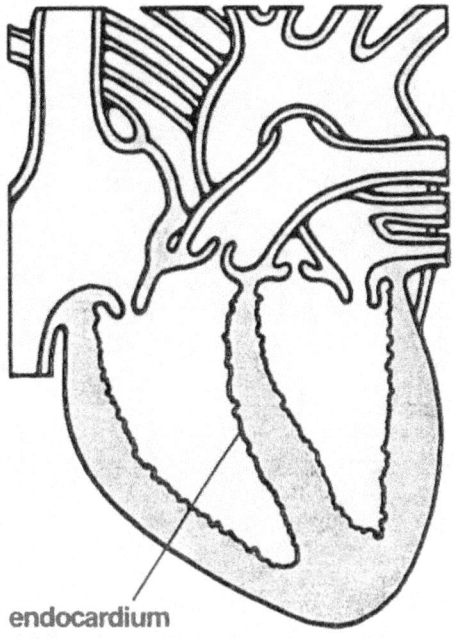

endocardium

ENDOMORPH *(en'do-morf)*
Short and thickset body type.

ENDOTHELIUM *(en"do-the'le-um)*
The thin lining of the blood vessels.

ENLARGED HEART
A state in which the heart is larger than normal. This may be due to heredity, a large amount of exercise over a period of time, or conditions which cause the heart to work harder—such as high blood pressure, obesity and defects of the heart or great vessels.

ENZYME *(en'zim)*
A complex organic substance which is capable of speeding up specific biochemical processes in the body. Enzymes are universally present in living organisms.

EPICARDIUM *(ep"e-kar'de-um)*
The outer layer of the heart wall. Also called the visceral pericardium.

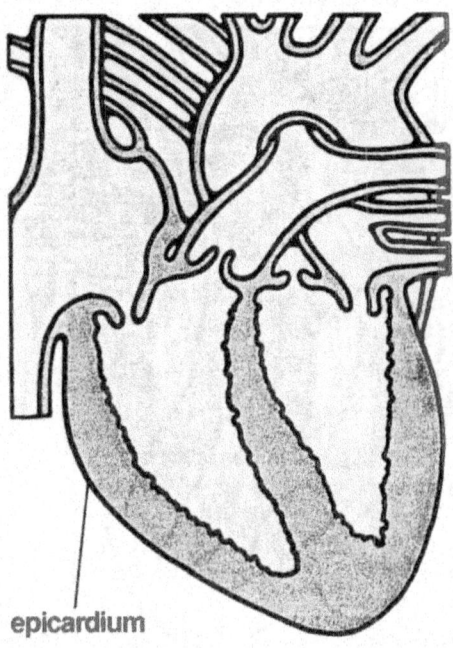
epicardium

EPIDEMIOLOGY *(ep'e-de"me-ol'-o-je)*
The science dealing with the factors which determine the frequency and distribution of a disease in a human community.

EPINEPHRINE *(ep"e-nef'rin)*
One of the secretions of two small glands, called adrenal glands, located just above the kidneys. This secretion, also called adrenalin, and sometimes prepared synthetically, constricts the small blood vessels (arterioles), increases the heart rate, and raises blood pressure. It is a vasoconstrictor or vasopressor substance.

ERYTHROCYTE *(e-rith'ro-site)*
Red blood cell.

ESOPHOGEAL VARICES *(e-sof"ah-je'al var'i-seez)*
Varicosed or swollen veins in the wall of the esophagus, the tube connecting the mouth and the stomach. These are dangerous because they may rupture and bleed profusely. Esophageal varices are often associated with cirrhosis of the liver. **See Varix.**

ESSENTIAL HYPERTENSION *(e-sen'shal hi"per-ten'shun)*
Sometimes called primary hypertension, and commonly known as high blood pressure. An elevated blood pressure of unknown cause.

ETIOLOGY *(e"te-ol'o-je)*
The sum of knowledge about the causes of a disease.

EXERCISE ELECTROCARDIOGRAM *(e-lek"tro-kar'de-o-gram")*
Often referred to as a "stress test." An electrocardiogram taken while the patient is exercising—usually jogging on a treadmill, walking up and down a short set of stairs, or pedaling on a stationary bicycle. **See Electrocardiogram.**

EXTRACORPOREAL CIRCULATION *(eks"trah-kor-po're-al)*
The circulation of the blood outside the body as by a mechanical pump or pump-oxygenator. This is often done while surgery is being performed on the heart.

EXTRASYSTOLE *(eks"trah-sis'to-le)*
A contraction of the heart which occurs prematurely and interrupts the normal rhythm.

EYEGROUND *(i'ground)*
The inside of the back part of the eye seen by looking through the pupil. Examining the eyeground is one means of assessing changes in the blood vessels. Also called fundus of the eye.

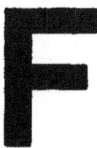

FABRICIUS AB AQUAPENDENTE, HIERONYMUS (1560-1634)
Italian anatomist, a teacher of William Harvey at Padua. He studied the valves of the veins. Harvey is reported to have credited the work of Fabricius with leading to his own concept of the circulation of the blood.

FALLOT, ETIENNE LOUIS ARTHUR (1850-1911) *(fal-o')*
French physician who gave an important description of a congenital heart defect known as the Tetralogy of Fallot (more accurately, *Tetrad* of Fallot). **See Tetralogy of Fallot.**

FEMORAL ARTERY *(fem'or-al ar'ter-e)*
Main blood vessel supplying blood to the leg.

FIBRILLATION *(fi-bri-la'shun)*
A kind of cardiac arrhythmia. Uncoordinated contraction of the heart muscle occurring when the individual muscle fibers take up independent irregular contractions. **Atrial fibrillation** involves very rapid, irregular contractions of the atria, followed irregularly by contractions of the ventricles. This may occur suddenly and for a short time, or, if there is an existing heart disease, can become chronic. Treatment is usually by drugs and sometimes by cardioversion (brief electric shock). **Ventricular fibrillation** involves contractions of the ventricles which are irregular, haphazard and ineffective, resulting in a rapid decline of blood circulation and death. Emergency treatment may include external cardiac massage (cardiopulmonary resuscitation—CPR), electrical defibrillation (cardioversion) or drugs. **See Cardiopulmonary Resuscitation and Cardioversion.**

FIBRIN *(fi'brin)*
An elastic, threadlike protein which forms the essential portion of a blood clot.

FIBRINOGEN *(fi-brin'o-jen)*
A protein dissolved in the blood which, by the action of certain enzymes, is converted into the insoluble threadlike protein of a blood clot (fibrin).

FIBRINOLYSIN *(fi"bri-no-li'sin)*
An enzyme which can cause coagulated blood to return to a liquid state.

FIBRINOLYTIC AGENTS *(fi"bri-no-lit'ik)*
Also called thrombolytic agents. Substances which dissolve blood clots. Two examples are streptokinase and urokinase.

FLOPPY MITRAL VALVE SYNDROME
See Barlow's Syndrome.

FLUORESCENT ANTIBODY TEST *(floo"o-res'ent an'te-bod"e)*
A rapid and sensitive laboratory test. Among other things, it can be used to detect the disease-causing bacteria known as streptococci, especially those that cause rheumatic fever and therefore rheumatic heart disease. The test consists of "tagging" with a fluorescent dye the antibodies, i.e., substances in blood serum that have been built up to defend the body against bacteria. This dyed antibody is then mixed with a smear taken from the throat of the patient. If there are streptococci present in the smear, the glowing antibodies will attach to them, and they can be clearly seen through a microscope. **See Rheumatic Fever and Rheumatic Heart Disease.**

FLUOROSCOPE *(floo'o-ro-skop)*
An instrument for observing the internal body organs at work. X-rays are passed through the body onto a fluorescent screen where the shadows of the beating heart and other organs can be seen and studied.

FLUOROSCOPY *(floo"or-os'ko-pe)*
The examination of structures within the body by means of a fluoroscope.

FLUTTER
See Atrial Flutter.

FORAMEN OVALE *(fo-ra'men o-va"le)*
An oval hole between the left and right upper chambers of the heart which normally closes shortly after birth. Its failure to close is one of the congenital defects of the heart, called a patent (open) foramen ovale.

FUNDUS OF THE EYE *(fun'dus)*
The inside of the back part of the eye seen by looking through the pupil. Examining the fundus of the eye is used as a means of assessing changes in the blood vessels. Also called the eyeground.

G

GALEN (CLAUDIUS GALENUS) (c. 130-200 A.D.)
Renowned Greek physician whose theory that life and health depended upon the balance of four "humors" in the body dominated medical practice for 1500 years. His concept of the ebb and flow of the blood (which transported the humors to various parts of the body) was not refuted until William Harvey's discovery of the circulation of the blood in 1628.

GALLOP RHYTHM
An extra heart sound which, when the heart rate is rapid enough, resembles a horse's gallop. It may or may not be significant.

GANGLION *(gang'gle-on)*
A mass of nerve cells which serves as a center of nervous influence.

GANGLIONIC BLOCKING AGENTS *(gang"gle-on'ik)*
Drugs which block the transmission of a nerve impulse at the nerve centers (ganglia) rather than at the nerve endings (as would adrenergic blocking agents). Some of these drugs, such as hexamethonium and mecamylamine hydrochloride, may be used in the treatment of high blood pressure.

GENETICS *(je-net'iks)*
The study of heredity.

GUANETHIDINE *(gwa-ne'thi-deen)*
One of the drugs used to control high blood pressure. **See Antihypertensive Drugs.**

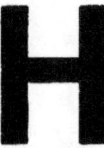

HARVEY, WILLIAM (1578-1657)
English physician who discovered the circulation of the blood and described his theory in 1628 in his classic work *De Motu Cordis*.

HEART ATTACK
The death of a portion of heart muscle which may result in disability or death of the individual, depending on how much of the heart is damaged. A heart attack occurs when an obstruction in one of the coronary arteries prevents an adequate oxygen supply to the heart. Symptoms may be none, mild or severe and may include chest pain (sometimes radiating to the shoulder, arm, neck or jaw), nausea, cold sweat, and shortness of breath.

Doctors often refer to a heart attack in terms of the obstruction (i.e., coronary occlusion, coronary thrombosis, or simply "coronary") or of the heart muscle damage (myocardial infarction, "infarct," or "M.I."). In common usage, the term "heart attack" often incorrectly refers to irregular heartbeats or attacks of angina pectoris.

HEART BLOCK
A condition in which the electrical impulse which travels through the heart's specialized conduction system to trigger the events of the heartbeat is slowed or blocked along its pathway. This can result in a dissociation of the rhythms of the upper and lower heart chambers, and is the major disorder for which artificial pacemakers are used. **See Sinoatrial Node and Pacemaker.**

HEART DISEASE
A general term used to mean ailments of the heart or blood vessels. Some of these are present at birth (congenital) and are either inherited or are the result of environmental influences on the embryo as it develops in the womb. The majority of cases of heart disease, however, are acquired later in life, for example, through the development of atherosclerosis.

HEART FAILURE
A condition in which the heart is unable to pump the amount of blood required to maintain a normal circulation. It can be isolated to either the left or the right side of the heart, or can involve the whole heart. Heart failure can develop from many heart and circulatory disorders, especially high blood pressure (an increased resistance to bloodflow in the arteries), heart attack, rheumatic heart disease and birth defects.

Heart failure often leads to congestion in the body tissues; fluid accumulates in the abdomen and legs and/or in the lungs (pulmonary edema). Congestive heart failure often develops gradually over several years, although it can be acute (short and severe). It can be treated by drugs or in some cases by surgery.

HEART-LUNG MACHINE
A machine through which the bloodstream is diverted for pumping and oxygenation, for example, during heart surgery. **See Extracorporeal Circulation.**

HEART MASSAGE
Also called cardiac massage. An emergency technique using compression of the heart to keep the blood pumping through the body in the event the heart stops pumping effectively. **External heart massage** involves pressing on the chest to compress the heart between the breastbone and the spine. Also, raising the pressure inside the chest by external compression may aid the heart's emptying as well. **Internal cardiac massage** is usually done in the operating room where the heart is directly compressed by the surgeon's hand through an incision in the chest.

HEMIPLEGIA *(hem"e-ple'je-ah)*
Paralysis of one side of the body caused by damage to the opposite side of the brain. Nerves cross in the brain, and one side of the brain controls the opposite side of the body. Such paralysis is sometimes caused by a blood clot or hemorrhage in a blood vessel in the brain. **See Stroke.**

HEMODYNAMICS *(he"mo-di-nam'iks)*
The study of the flow of blood and the forces involved.

HEMOGLOBIN *(he"mo-glo'bin)*
The oxygen-carrying red pigment of the red blood cells (corpuscles). When it has absorbed oxygen in the lungs, it is bright red and is called oxyhemoglobin. After it has given up some of its oxygen load in the tissues, it is dark burgundy in color and is called reduced hemoglobin.

HEMORRHAGE *(hem'or-ij)*
Loss of blood from a blood vessel. In external hemorrhage blood escapes from the body. In internal hemorrhage blood passes into tissues surrounding the ruptured blood vessel.

HEMORRHOIDS *(hem'o-roidz)*
Varices or excessively distended veins in the lower rectum and anus caused by a persistent increase in pressure within or against these veins. They are painful and often complicated by inflammation, bleeding, and clotting blood. **See Varix.**

HEPARIN *(hep'ah-rin)*
A naturally occurring substance which tends to prevent blood from clotting. Sometimes used in cases of an existing clot in an artery or vein to prevent enlargement of the clot or the formation of new clots. An anticoagulant.

HIGH BLOOD PRESSURE
An unstable or persistent elevation of blood pressure above the normal range. Uncontrolled, chronic high blood pressure strains the heart, damages arteries, and creates a greater risk of heart attack, stroke, and kidney problems. Also known as hypertension. **See Primary Hypertension and Secondary Hypertension.**

HIS, WILHELM (1831-1904) *(hiss)*
German anatomist who discovered the bundle of specialized muscle fibers running from the upper to lower chambers of the heart. These fibers are known as the "Bundle of His."

HYDRALAZINE *(hi-dral'ah-zeen)*
One of the drugs used to control high blood pressure. **See Antihypertensive Drugs.**

HYDROGENATED *(hi'dro-jen-a"tid)*
Combined with more hydrogen; more saturated.

HYPERCHOLESTEREMIA *(hi"per-ko-les"ter-e'me-ah)*
An excess of a fatty substance called cholesterol in the blood. Sometimes called hypercholesterolemia or hypercholesterinemia. **See Cholesterol.**

HYPERLIPEMIA *(hi"per-li-pe'me-ah)*
An excess of fats or lipids in the blood. Also called hyperlipidemia.

HYPERLIPOPROTEINEMIA *(hi"per-lip"o-pro"te-in-e'me-ah)*
The name for several types of blood-lipid disorders involving high blood levels of lipoproteins (complexes of lipids—either cholesterol or triglycerides—and certain kinds of proteins). Some types of hyperlipoproteinemia (Type II and Type IV) are associated with the premature development of atherosclerosis (hardening of the arteries) and therefore with increased risk of heart attack and stroke.

HYPERTENSION *(hi"per-ten'shun)*
Commonly called high blood pressure. **See High Blood Pressure, Primary Hypertension, and Secondary Hypertension.**

HYPERTENSIVE *(hi"per-ten'siv)*
A person with high blood pressure (hypertension).

HYPERTHYROIDISM *(hi"per-thi'roid-izm)*
A condition in which the thyroid gland is overly active. This may eventually result in a speeded up rate of heartbeat.

HYPERTROPHY *(hi-per'tro-fe)*
The enlargement of a tissue or organ due to increase in the size of its constituent cells. This may result from a demand for increased work.

HYPOCHOLESTEREMIC DRUGS *(hi"po-ko-les"te-re'mik)*
See Lipid-Lowering Drugs.

HYPOLIPEMIC DRUGS *(hi"po-li-pe'mik)*
Also called hypolipidemic drugs. **See Lipid-Lowering Drugs.**

HYPOTENSION *(hi"po-ten'shun)*
Commonly called low blood pressure. Blood pressure below the normal range. Most commonly used to describe an acute fall in blood pressure, as occurs in shock or syncope (fainting).

HYPOTHALAMUS *(hi"po-thal'ah-mus)*
A part of the brain which exerts control over activity of the abdominal organs, water balance, temperature, etc. Damage to the hypothalamus may cause abnormal gain in weight, among other things.

HYPOTHERMIA *(hy"po-ther'me-ah)*
Also called hypothermy. The state of low body temperature. Often induced (usually to 86-88 degrees F) during heart surgery in order to slow the metabolic processes. In this cooled state body tissues require less oxygen, and are therefore less likely to be damaged by oxygen deprivation.

HYPOTHYROIDISM *(hi"po-thi'roid-izm)*
A condition in which the thyroid gland is underactive, resulting in the slowing down of many of the body processes including the heart rate.

HYPOXIA *(hi-pok'se-ah)*
Less than normal content of oxygen in the organs and tissues of the body. At very high altitudes a healthy person experiences hypoxia because of insufficient oxygen in the air.

I

IATROGENIC HEART DISEASE *(i"at-ro-jen'ik)*
Literally means "caused by the doctor." A heart ailment inadvertently caused by the doctor or simply by the patient's belief that he has heart disease inferred from the manner and actions of his physician or other member of the medical team.

IDIOPATHIC HYPERTROPHIC SUBAORTIC STENOSIS (IHSS) *(id"e-o-path'ik hi"per-tro'fik sub"a-or'tik ste-no'sis)*
See Asymmetric Septal Hypertrophy.

ILIAC ARTERY *(il'e-ak ar'ter-e)*
A large artery which conducts blood to the pelvis and the legs.

INCIDENCE *(in'si-dens)*
The number of new cases of a disease developing in a given population during a specified period of time, such as a year.

INCOMPETENT VALVE *(in-kom'pe-tent)*
Any valve which does not close tight and leaks blood back in the wrong direction. Also called valvular insufficiency.

INFARCT *(in'farkt)*
The area of tissue which is damaged or dies as a result of receiving an insufficient blood supply. Frequently used in the phrase "myocardial infarct," referring to the area of heart muscle injury due to the interrupted flow of blood through the coronary artery which normally supplies it.

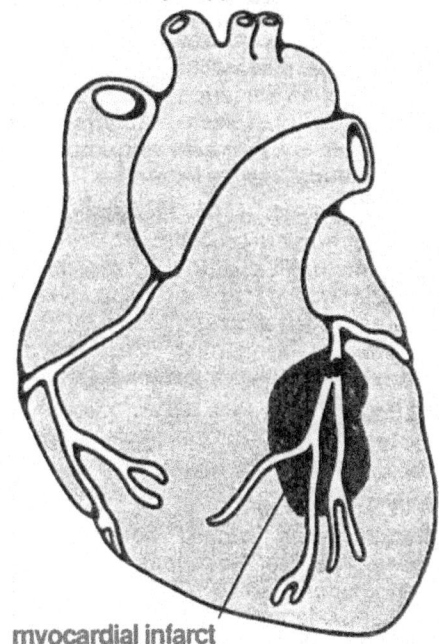

myocardial infarct

INFARCTION *(in-fark'shun)*
The occurrence of an infarct.

INNOMINATE ARTERY *(in-nom'i-nat)*
One of the largest branches of the aorta. It arises from the arch of the aorta and divides to form the right common carotid artery and the right subclavian artery.

INTERATRIAL SEPTUM *(in"ter-a'tre-al sep'tum)*
Sometimes called atrial septum. Muscular wall dividing left and right upper chambers (the atria) of the heart.
For illustration see Septum.

INTERMITTENT CLAUDICATION
(in"ter-mit'ent klaw"di-ka'shun)
Pain in the muscles of a limb which, similar to angina pectoris, occurs intermittently—during stress but not at rest. This condition frequently accompanies diseases of the peripheral blood vessels, such as thromboangiitis obliterans. The resting muscle has an adequate blood supply, but when the need for blood increases (as during exercise), the disease impairs the circulation. An inadequate blood supply and the buildup of waste products of metabolism in the tissues cause pain. "Claudication" means lameness.

INTERVENTRICULAR SEPTUM
(in"ter-ven-trik'u-lar sep'tum)
Sometimes called ventricular septum. Muscular wall, thinner at the top, dividing the left and right lower chambers of the heart which are called ventricles. **For illustration see Septum.**

INTIMA *(in'ti-mah)*
The innermost layer of a blood vessel (it includes the endothelium).

IN VITRO *(in vee'tro)*
Literally means "in glass," hence in a laboratory vessel. Describes a phenomenon studied outside a living body under laboratory conditions. **See In Vivo.**

IN VIVO *(in vee'vo)*
In a living organism. Describes a phenomenon studied in a living body. **See In Vitro.**

ISCHEMIA *(is-ke'me-ah)*
A local, usually temporary, deficiency of oxygen in some part of the body, often caused by a constriction or an obstruction in the blood vessel supplying that part.

ISCHEMIC HEART DISEASE *(is-kem'ik)*
Also called coronary artery disease and coronary heart disease. Heart ailments caused by narrowing of the coronary arteries and therefore a decreased blood supply to the heart (ischemia).

ISOPROTERENOL *(i"so-pro"te-re'nol)*
A drug which can be used as a cardiac stimulant to treat an abnormally slow heartbeat.

ISOTOPE *(i'so-top)*
Any of two or more species of a chemical element. The isotopes of one element are chemically identical, but differ by some physical property such as mass or radioactivity. Radioactive isotopes (radioisotopes) are often used in medicine to trace the fate of substances in the body. **See Radioisotopic Scanning.**

J

JUGULAR VEINS *(jug'u-lar)*
Veins which return blood from the head and neck to the heart.

L

LAENNEC, RENE THEOPHILE HYACINTHE (1781-1826)
French physician who invented the stethoscope.

LEEUWENHOEK, ANTONY VAN (1632-1723)
Dutch microscopist who, among other scientific contributions, discovered the interwoven structure of the muscle fibers of the heart.

LEUKOCYTES *(lu'ko-sitz)*
See White Blood Cells.

LIFESTYLE
An individual's typical way of life, including diet, kinds of recreation, job, home environment, location, temperament, and smoking, drinking and sleeping habits.

LINOLEIC ACID *(lin-o-lay'ik)*
An important component of many of the unsaturated fats. It is found widely in oils from plants. A diet with a high linoleic acid content tends to lower the amount of cholesterol in the blood.

LIPID *(lip'id)*
A fatty substance.

LIPID-LOWERING DRUGS
Drugs used to treat the various types of hyperlipoproteinemia, that is, abnormally high concentrations of lipids (fats) in the blood. Also called hypolipemic and hypolipidemic drugs; those drugs that lower blood levels of the lipid cholesterol are called hypocholesteremic.

The most common lipid-lowering drugs used are cholestyramine, clofibrate and nicotinic acid.

LIPOPROTEIN *(lip"o-pro'te-in)*
A complex consisting of lipid (fat) and protein molecules bound together. Lipids do not dissolve in the blood, but must circulate in the form of lipoproteins.

LUMEN *(lu'men)*
The passageway inside a tubular organ. The vascular lumen is the passageway inside a blood vessel.

M

MALIGNANT HYPERTENSION *(mah-lig'nant hi"per-ten'shun)*
Severe high blood pressure that may run a rapid course and cause damage to the blood vessel walls in the kidney, eye, and other organs. Its cardinal feature is central nervous system impairment, for example, coma, seizures, etc.

MALPIGHI, MARCELLO (1628-1694)
Italian anatomist who, among other discoveries, demonstrated the existence of capillary connections between the arteries and veins in the lungs.

MESOMORPH *(mes'o-morf)*
Muscular body type.

METABOLISM *(me-tab'o-lizm)*
A general term designating all chemical changes which occur to substances within the body.

METHYLDOPA *(meth"il-do'pah)*
One of the drugs used to control high blood pressure. **See Antihypertensive Drugs.**

MITRAL INSUFFICIENCY *(mi'tral in"su-fish'en-se)*
An incomplete closing of the mitral valve between the upper and lower chamber in the left side of the heart which permits a backflow of blood in the wrong direction. Sometimes the result of scar tissue forming after a rheumatic fever infection.

MITRAL STENOSIS *(mi'tral ste-no'sis)*
A narrowing of the valve (called the mitral valve) opening between the upper and lower chamber in the left side of the heart. Sometimes the result of scar tissue forming after a rheumatic fever infection.

MITRAL VALVE *(mi'tral)*
A valve of two cusps or triangular segments, located between the upper and lower chamber in the left side of the heart. **See Valve.**

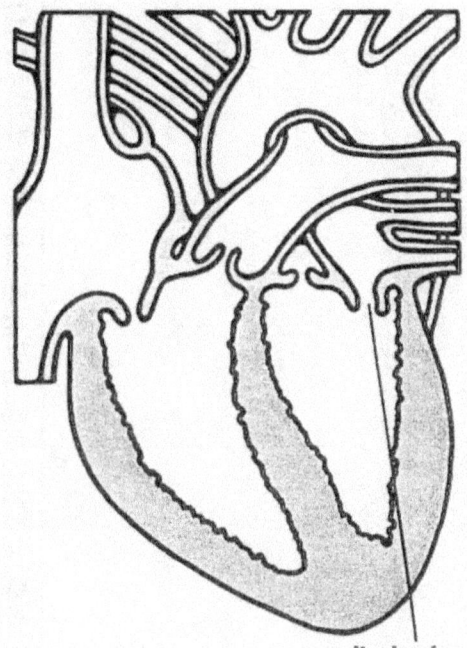

mitral valve

MITRAL VALVULOTOMY *(mi'tral val"vu-lot'o-me)*
An operation to widen the opening of the mitral valve by means of surgery with a knife. Usually performed when the valve opening is so narrowed as to obstruct bloodflow, which sometimes happens as a result of rheumatic fever. **See Commissurotomy.**

MONO-UNSATURATED FAT *(mon"o-un-sat'u-rat-ed)*
A fat so constituted chemically that it is capable of absorbing additional hydrogen but not as much hydrogen as polyunsaturated fat. These fats in the diet have little effect on the amount of cholesterol in the blood. One example is olive oil. **See Polyunsaturated Fat.**

MORBIDITY RATE *(mor-bid'i-te)*
The ratio of the number of **cases** of a disease to the number of **well people** in a given population during a specified period of time, such as a year. The term "morbidity" involves two separate concepts:
a. **Incidence** is the number of new cases of a disease developing in a given population during a specific period of time, such as a year.
b. **Prevalence** is the number of cases of a given disease existing in a given population at a specified moment of time.

MORTALITY RATE, AGE-ADJUSTED *(mor-tal'i-te)*
Also called age-adjusted death rate. Death rates which have been standardized for age for the purpose of making comparisons between different populations or within the same population at various intervals of time. The age-specific death rates of the populations being compared are applied to a population that is arbitrarily selected as standard, to determine what would be the crude death rate in the standard population if it were exposed first to the rates of one population and then to the rates of the other.

MORTALITY RATE, AGE-SPECIFIC *(mor-tal'i-te)*
Also called age-specific death rate. The ratio of deaths in a specific age group to the population of the same age group during a given period of time, such as a year. It is calculated by dividing the deaths that occurred among the specific age group during the year by the mid-year population in the same group (estimated population in the age group on July 1) of the same year.

MORTALITY RATE, CAUSE-SPECIFIC *(mor-tal'i-te)*
The ratio of deaths from a specific cause to total population during a given period of time, such as a year.

MORTALITY RATE, CRUDE *(mor-tal'i-te)*
The ratio of total deaths to total population during a given period of time, such as a year. Sometimes called crude death rate. It is calculated by dividing the total number of deaths during the year by the mid-year population (estimated population on July 1) of the same year.

MORTALITY RATE (SPECIFIC-CAUSE-OF-DEATH) *(mor-tal'i-te)*
The number of deaths from a specific cause that occurred in a unit of population (such as per 100,000 or per 10,000 or per 1,000) in a specified time, such as a year.

MURMUR *(mur'mur)*
An extra heart sound, sounding like fluid passing an obstruction, heard between the normal heart sounds.

MYOCARDIAL INFARCTION *(mi"o-kar'de-al in-fark'shun)*
The damaging and death of an area of heart muscle (myocardium) resulting from an interruption in the blood supply reaching that area. **See Heart Attack.**

MYOCARDITIS *(mi"o-kar-di'tis)*
Inflammation of the heart muscle (myocardium). It may be due to a variety of diseases, certain chemicals or drugs, trauma (e.g. electric shock or excessive x-ray treatment), or may be of unknown origin.

MYOCARDIUM *(mi"o-kar'de-um)*
The muscular wall of the heart. The thickest of the three layers of the heart wall, it lies between the inner layer (endocardium) and the outer layer (epicardium).

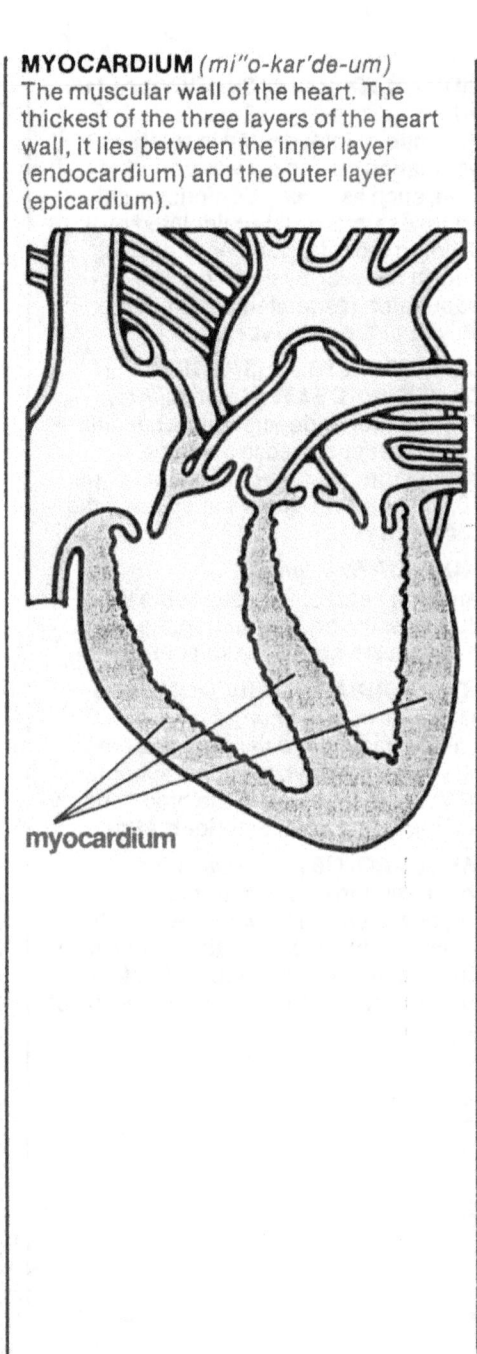

N

NEUROCIRCULATORY ASTHENIA (nu"ro-cir'cu-lah-to"re as-the'na-ah)
Sometimes called soldier's heart, effort syndrome, or functional heart disease. A complex of nervous and circulatory symptoms, often involving a sense of fatigue, dizziness, shortness of breath, rapid heartbeat, and nervousness. **See Effort Syndrome.**

NEUROGENIC (nu"ro-jen'ik)
Originating in the nervous system.

NICOTINIC ACID (nik'o-tin"ik)
A lipid-lowering drug which can be used to lower elevated levels of both cholesterol and triglycerides in the blood. **See Lipid-Lowering Drugs.**

NITRITES (ni'trits)
A group of chemical compounds, many of which cause dilation of the small blood vessels and thus lower blood pressure. Examples are amyl nitrite, sodium nitrite, nitroprusside and nitroglycerin.

NITROGLYCERIN (ni-tro-glis'er-in)
A drug (one of the nitrites) which relaxes the muscles in the blood vessels. Often used to relieve attacks of angina pectoris and spasm of coronary arteries. It is one of the vasodilators.

NORADRENALIN (nor"ad-ren'ah-lin)
See Norepinephrine.

NOREPINEPHRINE (nor"ep-e-nef'rin)
An organic compound which produces a rise in blood pressure by constricting the small blood vessels. Sometimes used in the treatment of shock. Also called noradrenalin.

NORMOTENSIVE (nor"mo-ten'siv)
Characterized by normal blood pressure.

NUTRITIONIST (nu-trish'un-ist)
One professionally engaged in investigating and solving problems of nutrition.

O

OBESITY (o-bees'i-te)
An increase in body weight beyond physical and skeletal requirements due to an accumulation of excess fat. This puts a strain on the heart and increases the chance of developing two major heart attack risk factors—high blood pressure and diabetes.

OCCLUSIVE (o-kloo'siv)
Closing or shutting off. A coronary occlusion is a closing off of a coronary artery (which supplies the heart muscle with blood).

OPEN-HEART SURGERY
Surgery performed on the opened heart. This phrase is also often used to refer to all heart surgery—whether or not the heart itself is opened.

ORGANIC HEART DISEASE
Heart disease caused by some structural abnormality in the heart or circulatory system.

OXYGEN (ok'si-jen)
A gas which is the most important component of the air we breathe. It is vital to energy-producing chemical reactions in the living cells of the body. Breathed into the lungs, it enters the bloodstream and is carried by the blood to the body tissues.

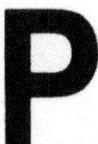

PACEMAKER *(pas'mak-er)*
A small mass of specialized cells in the right atrium of the heart which gives rise to the electrical impulses that initiate contractions of the heart. Also called sinoatrial node or S-A node of Keith-Flack. Under abnormal circumstances, other cardiac tissues may assume the pacemaker role by initiating electrical impulses which stimulate contraction.

The term "artifical pacemaker" is applied to an electrical device which can substitute for a defective natural pacemaker and control the beating of the heart by a series of rhythmic electrical discharges. If the electrodes which deliver the discharges to the heart are placed on the outside of the chest, it is called an "external pacemaker." If they are placed within the chest wall, it is called an "internal pacemaker."

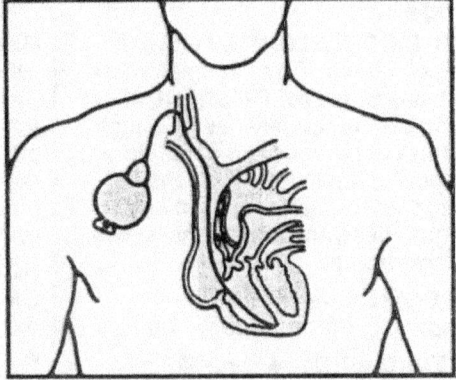

an implanted artificial pacemaker

PALPITATION *(pal"pi-ta'shun)*
A sensation of fluttering of the heart or abnormal rate or rhythm of the heart as experienced by the person.

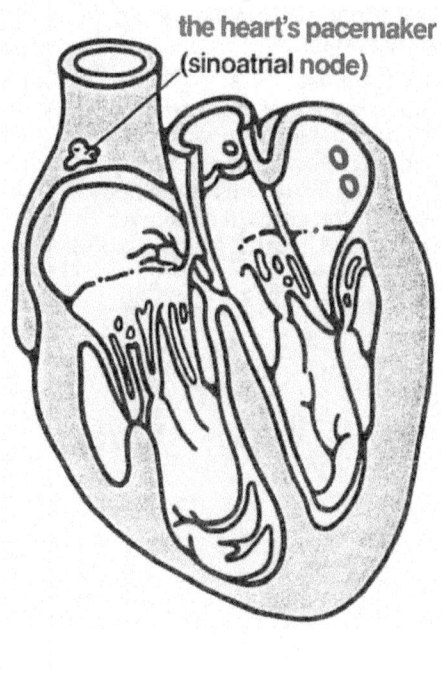

the heart's pacemaker (sinoatrial node)

PAPILLARY MUSCLES *(pap'i-ler"e)*
Small, cone-shaped muscles projecting from the walls of the lower heart chambers (the ventricles) to which are attached fibrous cords (chordae tendineae) stretching up to the flaps of the valves between upper and lower chambers. When the ventricles fill with blood and contract, the papillary muscles also contract and tighten the cords, allowing the valves to be pressed shut, but preventing them from being pushed back and open into the upper chambers (the atria) by the surging blood.

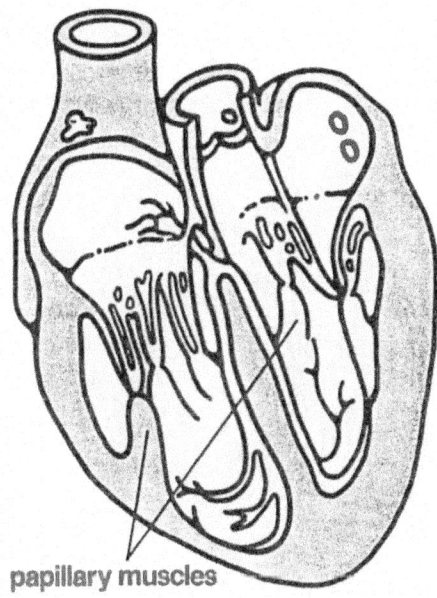

papillary muscles

PARASYMPATHETIC NERVOUS SYSTEM *(par"ah-sim"pah-thet'ik)*
One of the two divisions of the autonomic nervous system. **See Autonomic Nervous System.**

PARIETAL PERICARDIUM *(pah-ri'e-tal per"e-kar'de-um)*
A thickened protective membrane which is the outer wall of the pericardium, the double-walled sac surrounding the heart. **For illustration see Pericardium.**

PAROXYSMAL TACHYCARDIA *(par"ok-siz'mal tak"e-kar'de-ah)*
A period of rapid heartbeats which begins and ends suddenly.

PATENT DUCTUS ARTERIOSUS *(pa'tent duk'tus ar-te"re-o'sis)*
A congenital heart defect in which a small duct between the artery leaving the left side of the heart (aorta) and the artery leaving the right side of the heart (pulmonary artery), which normally closes soon after birth, remains open. As a result of this duct's failure to close, blood from both sides of the heart is pumped into the pulmonary artery and into the lungs. This defect is sometimes called simply patent ductus. Patent means open.

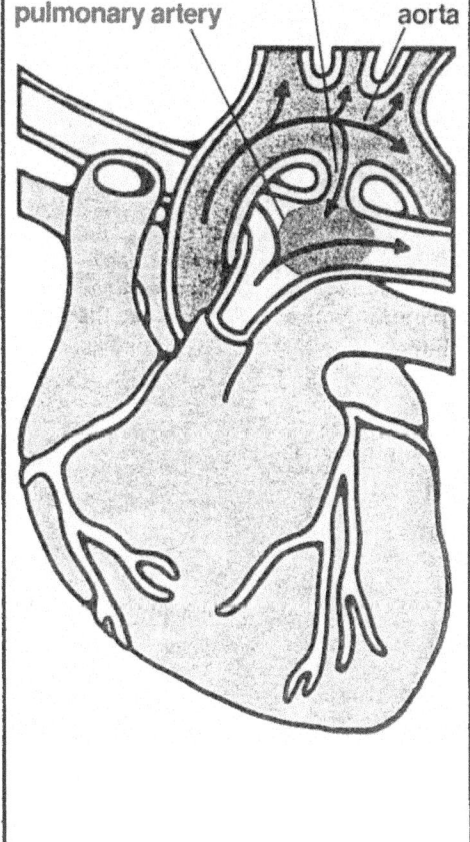

pulmonary artery — patent ductus arteriosus — aorta

PATENT FORAMEN OVALE *(pa'tent fo-ra'men o-va'le)*
One type of congenital heart defect. An oval hole (the foramen ovale) between the left and right upper chambers of the heart, which normally closes shortly after birth, remains open.

PERCUSSION *(per-kush'un)*
Tapping the body as an aid in diagnosing the conditions of parts beneath by the sound obtained. A physician will often tap the chest to determine the state of the heart and lungs—for instance, whether there may be a fluid accumulation or an enlarged heart.

PERIARTERITIS NODOSA *(per"e-ar"te-ri'tis no-do'sa)*
See Polyarteritis Nodosa.

PERICARDIAL TAMPONADE *(per"i-kar'de-al tam"pon-ad')*
An accumulation of excess fluid between the two layers of the membrane sac surrounding the heart (the pericardium). This can happen rapidly or gradually and impairs the normal functioning of the heart. **See Pericardium.**

PERICARDITIS *(per"e-kar-di'tis)*
Inflammation of the membrane sac (pericardium) which surrounds the heart.

PERICARDIUM *(per"e-kar'de-um)*
A closed sac surrounding the heart and roots of the great vessels. The sac is formed by two walls:
The **visceral pericardium** is on the inside, closely adhering to the heart. It forms the outermost layer of the heart wall and is also called the epicardium.
The **parietal pericardium** is on the outer side of the sac and is anchored to other chest structures such as the breastbone. It is a protective membrane.

The space inside the sac (the **pericardial cavity**), between the two walls, contains a fluid which provides for smooth movements of the heart as it beats.

PERIPHERAL RESISTANCE *(pe-rif'er-al)*
The resistance offered by the arterioles to the flow of blood. An increase in peripheral resistance causes a rise in blood pressure.

PERIPHERAL VASCULAR DISEASE (pe-rif'er-al vas'cu-lar)
A term which, in its broadest sense, refers to diseases of any of the blood vessels outside of the heart and to diseases of the lymph vessels. These are circulation disorders caused by changes in the caliber of the vessels. **Functional** peripheral vascular diseases are not structural or organic in cause, but are transient and reversible. An example is Raynaud's disease, which can be triggered by cold temperatures, emotional stress, work with vibrating machinery or smoking. The term **organic** describes circulation disturbances which are caused by structural changes in the vessels (such as inflammation and tissue damage). An example is Buerger's disease (thromboangiitis obliterans).

PERSONALITY, TYPE A AND TYPE B
See Behavior, Type A and Type B.

PHEOCHROMOCYTOMA (fe-o-kro"mo-si-to'mah)
A tumor which arises in the adrenal glands. It produces and releases into the bloodstream large quantities of norepinephrine and epinephrine. These powerful natural stimulants may then create such symptoms as high blood pressure, elevated heart rate, headaches, anxiety, and excessive sweating.

PHLEBITIS (fle-bi'tis)
Inflammation of a vein, often in the leg. Sometimes a blood clot is formed in the inflamed leg. **See also Thrombophlebitis.**

PHOSPHOLIPIDS (fos"fo-lip'idz)
One of the three major classes of lipids (fatty substances) in the blood. Unlike the other two classes—cholesterol and triglycerides—phospholipids are *not* known to be associated with atherosclerosis (hardening of the arteries).

PLAQUE (plak)
See Atheroma.

PLASMA (plaz'mah)
The cell-free liquid portion of uncoagulated blood. It is different from serum which is the fluid portion of the blood obtained after coagulation.

PLATELETS (plat'letz)
One of the three kinds of formed elements found in the blood. Literally "little plates," they are small, colorless, disk-shaped bodies which are involved in the formation of blood clots. Also called thrombocytes. **See Red Blood Cells and White Blood Cells.**

PLETHYSMOGRAPHY (pleth"iz-mog'rah-fe)
The recording of changes in the size of an organ, part, or limb as blood circulates through it. However, lung volumes can also be measured with the technique.

POLYARTERITIS NODOSA (pol"e-ar"te-ri'tis no-do'sa)
A disease of unknown cause characterized by inflammation and destruction along segments of small and medium-sized arteries, creating lumps or nodes of scar tissue. This leads to functional impairment of the tissues supplied by the affected vessels.

POLYCYTHEMIA (pol"e-si-the'me-ah)
An abnormal condition of the blood characterized by an excessive number of red blood cells.

POLYUNSATURATED FAT (pol"e-un-sat'u-rat-ed)
A fat so constituted chemically that it is capable of absorbing additional hydrogen. These fats are usually liquid oils of vegetable origin, such as corn oil or safflower oil. A diet with a high polyunsaturated fat content tends to lower the amount of cholesterol in the blood. These fats are sometimes substituted for saturated fat in a diet in an effort to lessen the hazard of fatty deposits in the blood vessels. **See Mono-unsaturated Fat.**

PRESSOR *(pres'or)*
Tending to increase blood pressure, as a pressor substance.

PREVALENCE *(prev'ah-lens)*
The number of cases of a given disease existing in a given population at a specified moment of time.

PRIMARY HYPERTENSION *(hi"per-ten'shun)*
Also called essential hypertension. High blood pressure of unknown origin (as opposed to secondary hypertension, which is caused by some primary disease, such as kidney disease). Most people who have high blood pressure have primary hypertension. **See Secondary Hypertension.**

PROCAINE AMIDE *(pro'kane am'id)*
A drug sometimes used to treat abnormal rhythms of the heartbeat; an antiarrhythmic drug.

PROPRANOLOL *(pro-pran'o-lol)*
A member of the group of drugs known as beta-blocking agents. Propranolol is used to treat angina pectoris, cardiac arrhythmias, high blood pressure, and other disorders of the cardiovascular system. **See Adrenergic Blocking Agents.**

PROSTAGLANDINS *(pros"tah-glan'dinz)*
Hormone-like substances made from fatty acids which are found throughout the body tissues. They are thought to have important roles in tissue metabolism and bloodflow, among other things.

PROSTHESIS *(pros-the'sis)*
An artificial substitute for a body part, such as a leg, tooth, heart valve or blood vessel. The plural form is **Prostheses.**

PSYCHOSOMATIC *(si"ko-so-mat'ik)*
Pertaining to the influence of the mind, emotions, fears, etc., upon the functions of the body, especially in relation to disease.

PULMONARY *(pul'mo-ner"e)*
Pertaining to the lungs.

PULMONARY ARTERY
The large artery which conveys unoxygenated (venous) blood from the lower right chamber of the heart to the lungs. This is the only artery in the body which normally carries unoxygenated blood, all others carrying oxygenated blood to the body.

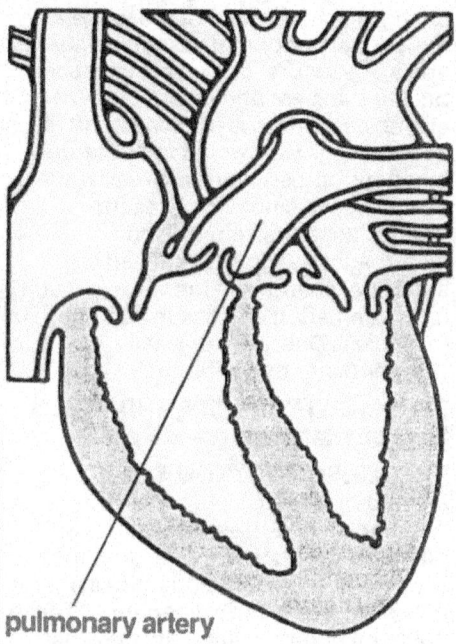

pulmonary artery

PULMONARY CIRCULATION
The circulation of the blood through the lungs, the flow being from the right lower chamber of the heart (right ventricle) through the lungs, back to the left upper chamber of the heart (left atrium). **See Systemic Circulation.**

PULMONARY EDEMA *(pul'mo-ner"e e-de'mah)*
A condition, usually acute (sudden and severe) but sometimes chronic, marked by an excess of fluid in the extravascular (outside the vessels) spaces in the lungs. It may be confined to the interstitial spaces or may appear in the alveoli (the millions of tiny air sacs in each lung). Pulmonary edema occurs most often as a complication of left ventricular failure due to ischemic heart disease, high blood pressure or disease of the aortic valve. **See Congestive Heart Failure and Heart Failure.**

PULMONARY EMBOLISM *(em'bo-lizm)*
A condition in which a blood clot (embolus), usually one formed in a vein of the leg or pelvis, breaks loose and becomes lodged in one of the arteries of the lungs. This may produce no symptoms at all or may create very serious impairment of pulmonary circulation.

PULMONARY HYPERTENSION *(hi"per-ten'shun)*
High blood pressure (hypertension) in the blood vessels of the lungs. The two most common causes are chronic obstructive lung diseases (such as emphysema) and septal defects (holes in the wall which separates the left and right sides of the heart).

PULMONARY VALVE
Valve formed by three cup-shaped membranes at the junction of the pulmonary artery and the right lower chamber of the heart (right ventricle). When the right ventricle contracts, the pulmonary valve opens and the blood is forced into the artery leading to the lungs. When the chamber relaxes, the valve is closed and prevents a backflow of the blood. **See Valve.**

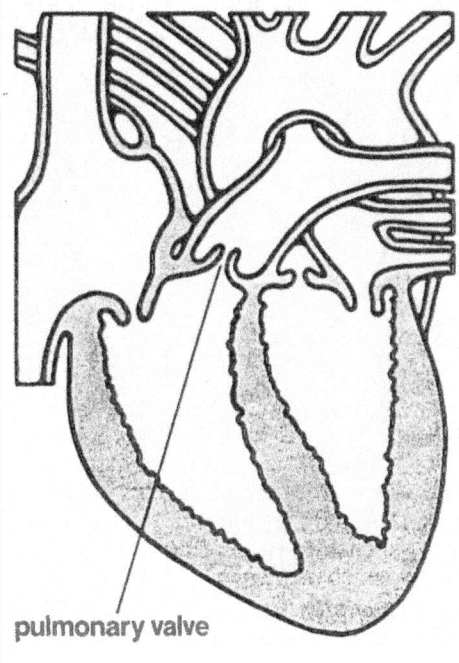
pulmonary valve

Q

PULMONARY VEINS
The veins which conduct oxygenated blood from the lungs into the left upper chamber of the heart (left atrium).

pulmonary veins   pulmonary veins

PULSE *(puls)*
The expansion and contraction of an artery which may be felt with the finger.

PULSE PRESSURE
The difference between the blood pressure in the arteries when the heart is in contraction (systole) and when it is in relaxation (diastole).

PULSUS ALTERNANS *(pul'sus awl-ter'nanz)*
A pulse in which there is regular alternation of weak and strong beats.

PURKINJE FIBERS *(pur-kin'je)*
Specialized muscular fibers forming a network in the walls of the lower chambers of the heart and believed to be involved in conducting electrical impulses to the muscular walls of the two lower chambers (ventricles). These electrical impulses are responsible for the contractions of the heart.

QUINIDINE *(kwin'i-deen)*
A drug sometimes used to treat abnormal rhythms of the heartbeat; an antiarrhythmic drug.

R

RADIOISOTOPE *(ray"de-o-i'so-top)*
A radioactive form ("isotope") of an element. **See Isotope.**

RADIOISOTOPIC SCANNING *(ray"de-o-i'so-top-ik skan'ning)*
A diagnostic technique involving radioactive labelling of tissues and organs by the injection of radioisotopes into the bloodstream. The emitted radioactivity is detected by a scanner and a record or "scan" of the labelled area is made. Used by cardiologists to visualize the heart and great vessels, it can often reveal areas of heart damage. **See Isotope and Radioisotope.**

RAUWOLFIA *(raw-wol'fe-ah)*
A drug consisting of powdered whole root of a plant (Rauwolfia serpentina) which lowers blood pressure and slows the heart rate. Sometimes used in treatment of high blood pressure. An antihypertensive agent. **See Reserpine.**

RAYNAUD'S DISEASE *(ray-noz')*
Also called Primary Raynaud's Phenomenon. A disorder characterized by occurrences of Raynaud's Phenomenon, but not known to have an underlying cause.

RAYNAUD'S PHENOMENON *(ray-noz')*
Short episodes of pallor and numbness in the fingers, toes and, rarely, the nose and ears, due to temporary constriction of the arterioles in the skin. Pallor in the affected area is followed by blueness (due to insufficient oxygen supply), then occasionally by redness as oxygenated blood rushes in. These episodes may be triggered by cold temperatures, emotional stress, working with vibrating machinery or cigarettes.

Primary Raynaud's Phenomenon is called **Raynaud's Disease**, is generally benign, and has no known cause.
Secondary Raynaud's Phenomenon is a symptom of one of several serious disorders, which, if not detected and treated, may have serious consequences.

RED BLOOD CELLS (CORPUSCLES)
One of the three kinds of formed elements found in the blood. Their most important function is to carry oxygen by means of hemoglobin, the red pigment these cells contain. Also called erythrocytes. **See White Blood Cells and Platelets.**

REGURGITATION *(re-gur"ji-ta'shun)*
The backward flow of blood through a defective valve.

REHABILITATION *(re"hah-bil"i-ta'shun)*
The return of a person disabled by accident or disease to the maximum attainable physical, mental, emotional, social and economic usefulness, and, if employable, to an opportunity for gainful employment.

RENAL *(re'nal)*
Pertaining to the kidney.

RENAL CIRCULATION
The circulation of the blood through the kidneys. Important in heart disease because of its functon in the elimination of water, certain chemical elements, and waste products from the body.

RENAL HYPERTENSION *(re'nal hi"per-ten'shun)*
High blood pressure caused by damage to or disease of the kidneys or their blood vessels.

RESERPINE *(res'er-peen OR re-ser'peen)*
One of the organic substances found in the root of the Indian snake root plant (Rauwolfia serpentina) which lowers blood pressure, slows the heart rate, and has a sedative effect.

REVASCULARIZATION *(re-vas"ku-lar-i-za'shun)*
Restoration of sufficient bloodflow to body tissues when supplying arteries are narrowed or blocked by injury or disease. Such surgery can be done on the legs, kidneys, brain, neck or (most commonly) the heart.

One procedure for cardiac revascularization is endarterectomy, removal of the thickened inner lining of a narrowed coronary artery. Other procedures may involve the use of additional blood vessels, either artificial ones or ones from elsewhere in the body. Vessels from other parts of the body may either be rerouted from nearby structures (for example, the internal mammary artery) or by grafting whole sections of vessels onto the heart (as is done with the saphenous vein in coronary bypass surgery). **See Endarterectomy and Coronary Bypass Surgery.**

RHEUMATIC FEVER *(roo-mat'ik)*
A disease, usually occurring in childhood, which may follow a few weeks after a streptococcal infection. It is sometimes characterized by one or more of the following: fever, sore swollen joints, a skin rash, occasionally by involuntary twitching of the muscles (called chorea or St. Vitus Dance) and small nodes under the skin. In some cases the infection affects the heart and may result in scarring the valves, weakening the heart muscle, or damaging the sac enclosing the heart. **See Rheumatic Heart Disease.**

RHEUMATIC HEART DISEASE *(roo-mat'ik)*
The damage done to the heart, particularly the heart valves, by one or more attacks of rheumatic fever. The valves are sometimes scarred so they do not open and close normally. **See Rheumatic Fever.**

RISK FACTORS
In cardiology, characteristics which are associated with an increased risk of developing coronary heart disease. These include high blood pressure (hypertension), elevated blood levels of cholesterol and other lipids (hyperlipoproteinemia), cigarette smoking, obesity, diabetes and a family history of heart disease. A competitive, aggressive lifestyle (Type A Behavior) is also thought to predispose a person to heart disease.

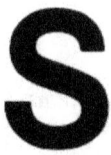

S-A NODE
See Sinoatrial Node.

SAPHENOUS VEIN (sah-fe'nus)
A large vein in the leg which can be removed and grafted onto the heart in coronary bypass surgery to provide adequate coronary circulation. **See Coronary Bypass Surgery.**

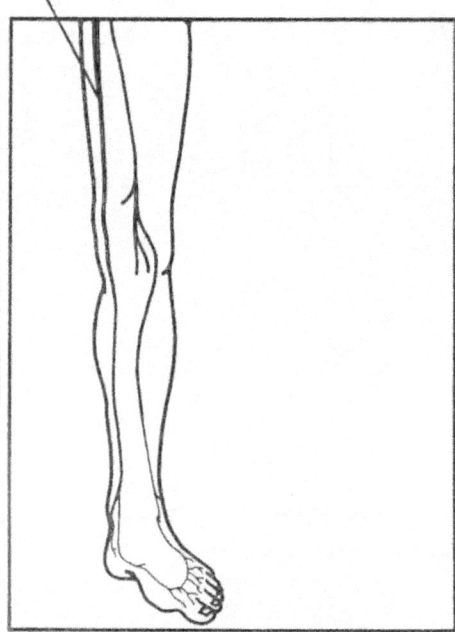

saphenous vein

SATURATED FAT (sat'u-rat"ed)
A fat so constituted chemically that it is not capable of absorbing any more hydrogen. These are usually the solid fats of animal origin such as the fats in milk, butter, meat, etc. A diet high in saturated fat content tends to increase the amount of cholesterol in the blood. Sometimes these fats are restricted in the diet in an effort to lessen the hazard of fatty deposits in the blood vessels.

SCLEROSIS (skle-ro'sis)
Hardening, as in the term "arteriosclerosis," hardening of the arteries.

SECONDARY HYPERTENSION (hi"per-ten'shun)
High blood pressure caused by (i.e. secondary to) certain specific diseases or infections. **See Pheochromocytoma and Renal Hypertension.**

SEMILUNAR VALVES (sem"e-lu'nar)
Cup-shaped valves. The aortic valve at the entrance to the aorta and the pulmonary valve at the entrance to the pulmonary artery are semilunar valves. They consist of three cup-shaped flaps which prevent the backflow of blood.

SEPTAL DEFECT (sep'tal)
An abnormal opening in the wall (septum) that normally divides the right and left sides of the heart. There are both atrial and ventricular septal defects, depending on whether the upper or lower heart chambers are involved.

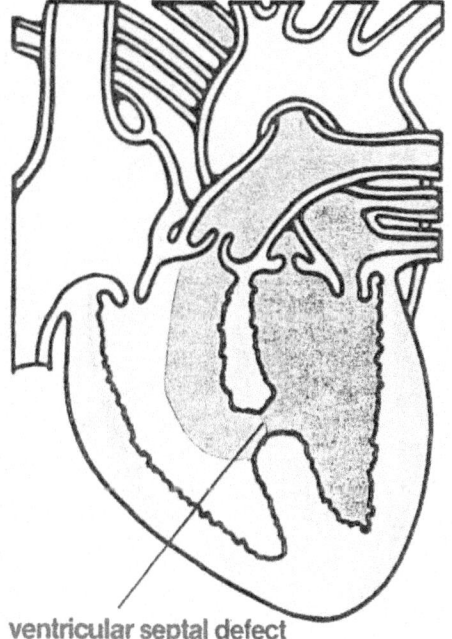

ventricular septal defect

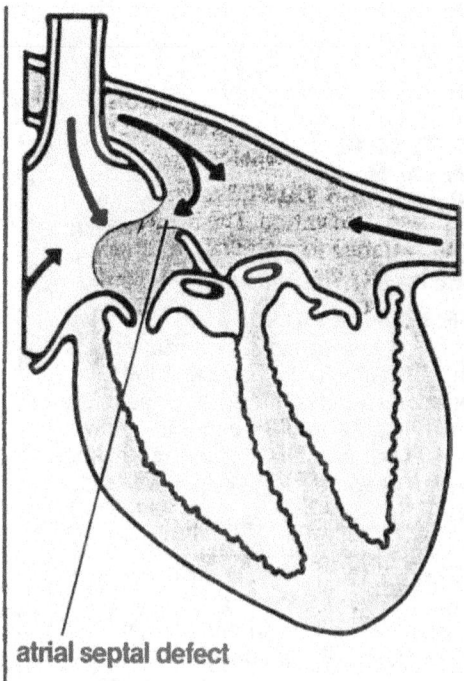

atrial septal defect

SEPTUM *(sep'tum)*
A dividing wall.
1. Atrial or interatrial septum. Muscular wall dividing left and right upper chambers (atria) of the heart.
2. Ventricular or interventricular septum. Muscular wall, thinner at the top, dividing the left and right lower chambers (ventricles) of the heart.

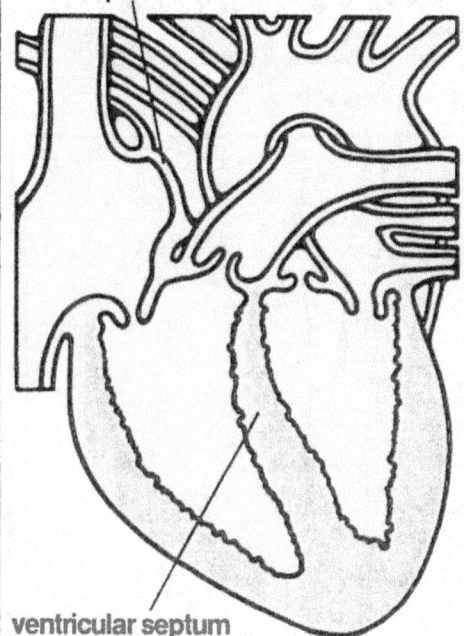

atrial septum

ventricular septum

SEROTONIN *(ser"o-to'nin)*
A naturally occurring compound, found mainly in the gastrointestinal tract and in lesser amounts in the blood, which has a stimulating effect on the circulatory system.

SERUM *(se'rum)*
The fluid portion of blood which remains after the cellular elements have been removed by coagulation. It is different from plasma which is the cell-free liquid portion of uncoagulated blood.

SERVETUS, MICHAEL (1509-1553)
Spanish physician who discovered the circulation of the blood through the lungs. Burned at the stake in Geneva for his religious doctrines.

SHOCK
The collection of symptoms resulting from an inadequate volume of fluid circulating through the body to maintain normal metabolism. This may be due to a large loss of blood or to some derangement of circulatory control. Shock is marked by hypotension (low blood pressure), pale, cold skin, usually tachycardia (weak, rapid pulse), and often anxiety. Cardiogenic shock is shock resulting from a greatly diminished cardiac output, such as may occur in a large heart attack.

SHUNT
A passage between two blood vessels or between the two sides of the heart, as in cases where an opening exists in the wall which normally separates them. In surgery, the operation of forming a passage between blood vessels to divert blood from one part of the body to another.

SIGN
Any objective evidence of a disease.
See Symptom.

SINOATRIAL NODE *(si"no-a'tre-al)*
A small mass of specialized cells in the right upper chamber of the heart which give rise to the electrical impulses that initiate contractions of the heart. Also called S-A node or pacemaker. **For illustration see Pacemaker.**

SINUS RHYTHM *(si'nus rith'm)*
Normal heart rhythm as initiated by electrical impulses in the sinoatrial node or pacemaker. **See Pacemaker.**

SINUSES OF VALSALVA *(si'nus-sez of val-sal'vah)*
Three pouches in the wall of the aorta behind the three cup-shaped membranes of the aortic valve.

SODIUM *(so'de-um)*
A mineral essential to life, found in nearly all plant and animal tissue. Table salt (sodium chloride) is nearly half sodium. In some types of heart disease the body retains an excess of sodium and water, and therefore sodium intake is restricted.

SPHYGMOMANOMETER *(sfig"mo-mah-nom'e-ter)*
An instrument for measuring blood pressure in the arteries.

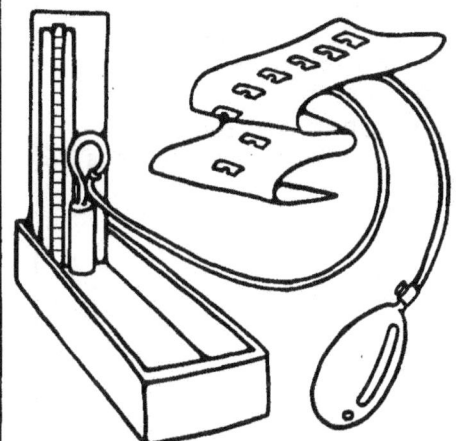

mercury column sphygmomanometer

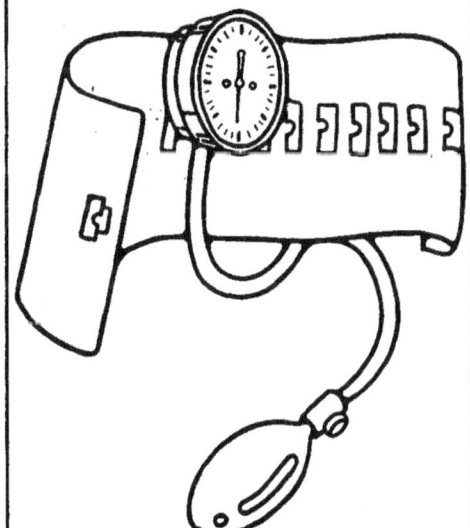

dial or aneroid sphygmomanometer

STARLING'S LAW OF THE HEART
A law which states that the more the heart muscle is stretched when an increased amount of blood fills the ventricles, the more vigorous its contraction will be, resulting in a greater amount of blood pumped out of the heart.

STASIS *(sta'sis)*
A stoppage or lessening of the flow of blood or other body fluid in any part.

STENOSIS *(ste-no'sis)*
A narrowing or stricture of an opening. Mitral stenosis, aortic stenosis, etc., mean that the valve indicated has become so narrowed that it does not function normally.

STETHOSCOPE *(steth'o-skop)*
An instrument for listening to sounds within the body.

STRESS
Bodily or mental tension caused by physical, chemical or emotional factors. Stress can refer to physical exertion as well as mental anxiety.

STRESS TEST
A diagnostic method used to determine the body's response to physical exertion (stress). Usually involves taking an ECG and other physiological measurements (such as breathing rate and blood pressure) while the patient is exercising—usually jogging on a treadmill, walking up and down a short set of stairs, or pedaling on a stationary bicycle.

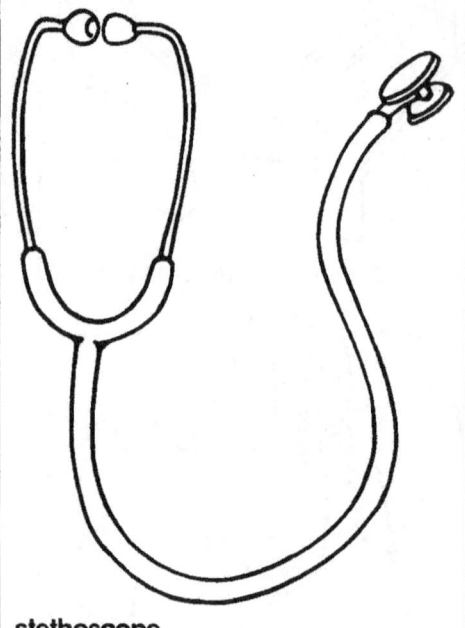

stethoscope

STROKE *(strok)*
Also called cerebral vascular accident. An impeded blood supply to some part of the brain, generally caused by:
1. A blood clot forming in the vessel (cerebral thrombosis).
2. A rupture of the blood vessel wall (cerebral hemorrhage).
3. A blood clot or other material from another part of the vascular system which flows to the brain and obstructs a cerebral vessel (cerebral embolism).
4. Pressure on a blood vessel, as by a tumor.

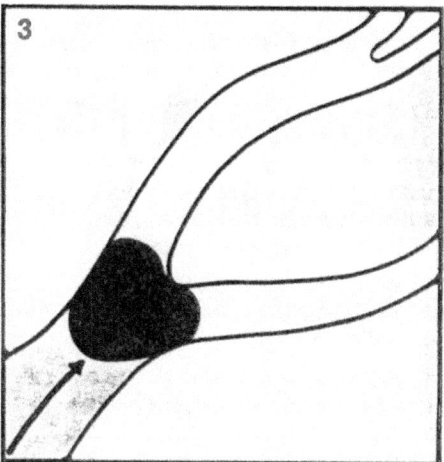

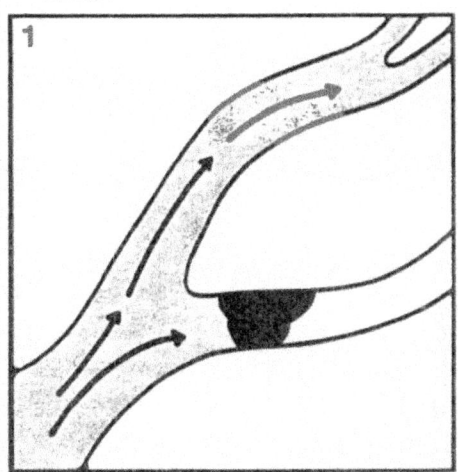

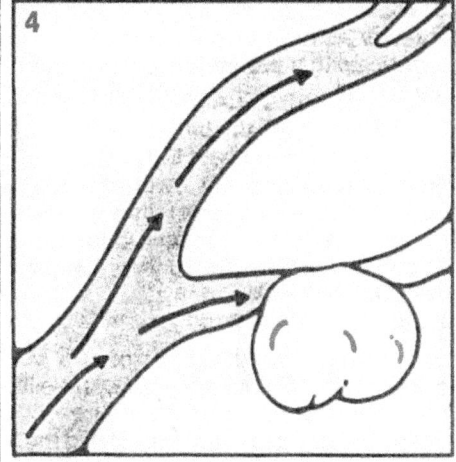

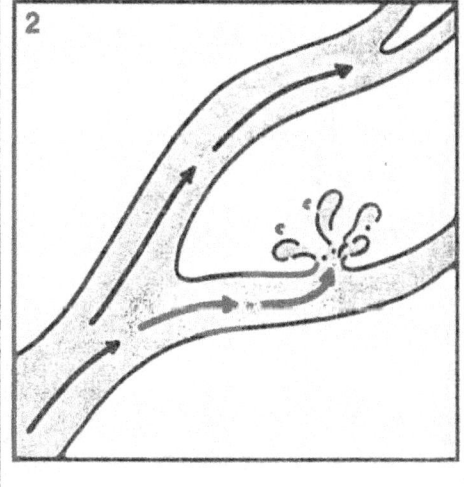

STROKE VOLUME *(strok)*
The amount of blood which is pumped out of the heart at each contraction of the heart.

SYMPATHECTOMY *(sim"pah-thek'to-me)*
An operation which interrupts some part of the sympathetic nervous system. The sympathetic nervous system is a part of the autonomic or involuntary nervous system which normally regulates tissues not under voluntary control, e.g., glands, heart, and smooth

muscles. Sometimes the interruption is accomplished by drugs, in which case it is called a chemical sympathectomy.

SYMPATHETIC NERVOUS SYSTEM *(sim"pah-thet'ik)*
One of the two divisions of the autonomic nervous system. **See Autonomic Nervous System.**

SYMPTOM *(simp'tum)*
Any subjective evidence of a patient's condition. **See Sign.**

SYNCOPE *(sin'ko-pe)*
A faint. One cause for syncope can be an insufficient blood supply to the brain.

SYNDROME *(sin'drom)*
A set of symptoms which occur together and are therefore given a name to indicate that particular combination.

SYSTEMIC CIRCULATION *(sis-tem'ik)*
The circulation of the blood through all parts of the body except the lungs, the flow being from the left lower chamber of the heart (left ventricle) through the body, back to the right upper chamber of the heart (right atrium). **See Pulmonary Circulation.**

SYSTOLE *(sis'to-le)*
In each heartbeat, the period of contraction of the heart. Atrial systole is the period of the contraction of the upper chambers of the heart, called the atria.

Ventricular systole is the period of the contraction of the lower chambers of the heart, called the ventricles. **See Cardiac Cycle.**

T

TACHYCARDIA *(tak"e-kar'de-ah)*
Abnormally fast heart rate. Generally, anything over 100 beats per minute is considered a tachycardia.

TETRALOGY OF FALLOT *(te-tral'o-je of fal-o')*
A congenital malformation of the heart involving four distinct defects (hence tetralogy). Named for Etienne Fallot, French physician who described the condition in 1888. The four defects are:
1. An abnormal opening in the wall between the lower chambers of the heart (ventricular septal defect).
2. Misplacement of the aorta, "overriding" the abnormal opening, so that is receives blood from both the right and left lower chambers instead of only the left.
3. Pulmonary outflow obstruction usually below or at the valve.
4. Enlargement of the right ventricle.

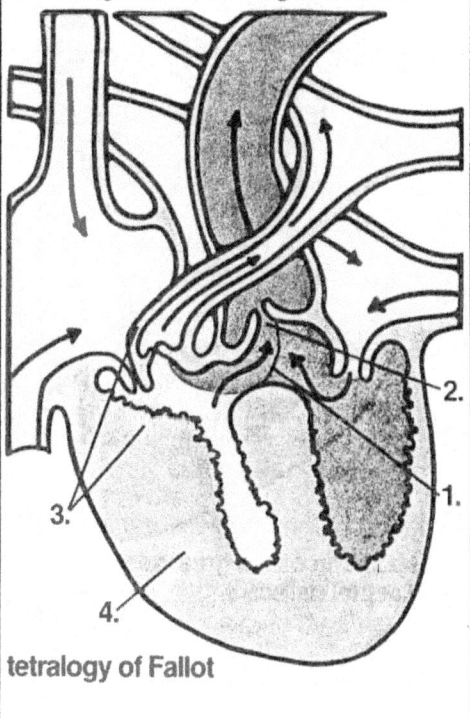

tetralogy of Fallot

THIAZIDES *(thi'a-sidz)*
Also called thiazide diuretics or benzothiadiazides. A class of diuretics (drugs which promote excretion of urine) which includes chlorothiazide. The thiazides are often used to treat high blood pressure and for the relief of edema, or waterlogged tissues. **See Antihypertensive Drugs.**

THORACIC *(tho-ras'ik)*
Pertaining to the chest (thorax).

THROMBECTOMY *(throm-bek'to-me)*
An operation to remove a blood clot from a blood vessel.

THROMBOANGIITIS OBLITERANS *(throm"bo-an"je-i'tis ob-lit'er-anz)*
Also called Buerger's disease. A disease of the blood vessels of the extremities, primarily the legs, which occurs most commonly in men and is associated with tobacco use. It is characterized by inflammation of the veins, arteries and nerves and by thrombosis in the vessels (blood clot formation). This leads to poor circulation and gangrene. **See Buerger's Syndrome.**

THROMBOEMBOLISM *(throm"bo-em'bo-lizm)*
Obstruction (embolism) of a blood vessel by a blood clot (thrombus) formed elsewhere in the circulatory system and carried along by the bloodstream to plug a smaller vessel.

THROMBOLYTIC AGENTS *(throm"bo-lit'ik)*
Substances which dissolve blood clots. Also called fibrinolytic agents. Two examples are streptokinase and urokinase.

THROMBOPHLEBITIS *(throm"bo-fle-bi'tis)*
Inflammation and blood clotting in a vein.

THROMBOSIS *(throm-bo'sis)*
The formation or presence of a blood clot (thrombus) inside a blood vessel or cavity of the heart.

THROMBUS *(throm'bus)*
A blood clot which forms inside a blood vessel or cavity of the heart. **See Embolus.**

TOXIC *(tok'sik)*
Poisonous,

TRANSPLANTATION, HEART
The replacement of a healthy heart from a recently deceased donor into the chest of a person whose own heart can no longer function adequately. The donor's heart then replaces or assists the failing heart.

TRANSPOSITION OF THE GREAT VESSELS *(trans"po-zish'un)*
A congenital heart defect in which the two largest arteries occur in the wrong places: the aorta arises from the right (rather than left) ventricle and the pulmonary artery arises from the left (rather than right) ventricle. Thus the right heart pumps used blood from the body through the aorta and back to the body, and the left heart pumps oxygenated blood from the lungs back to the lungs. Only if there is a sizeable hole between right and left chambers.(a septal defect) or a channel between the aorta and pulmonary artery (patent ductus arteriosus) will enough oxygenated blood get pumped to the body to sustain life for the infant.

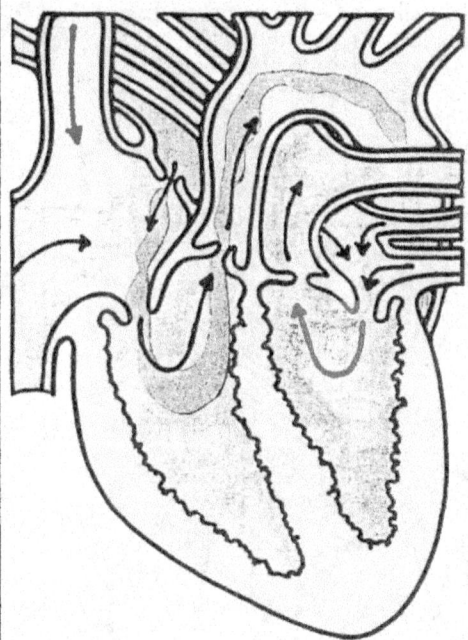

transposition of the great vessels with atrial septal defect

TRICUSPID VALVE *(tri-kus'pid)*
A valve consisting of three cusps or triangular segments located between the upper and lower chamber in the right side of the heart. Its position corresponds to the mitral valve (which is bicuspid) in the left side of the heart. **See Valve.**

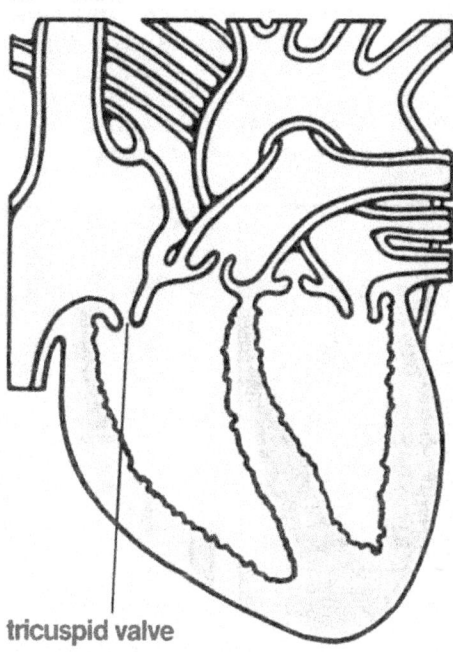

tricuspid valve

TRIGLYCERIDE *(tri-glis'er-id)*
The main type of lipid (fatty substance) found in the adipose (fat) tissue of the body and also the main dietary lipid. High levels of triglycerides in the blood may be associated with a greater risk of coronary atherosclerosis.

TRUNCUS ARTERIOSUS *(trun'kus ar-te"re-o'sus)*
An arterial trunk arising from the fetal heart which develops into the aorta and pulmonary artery. It is a congenital defect if it persists past the birth of the infant.

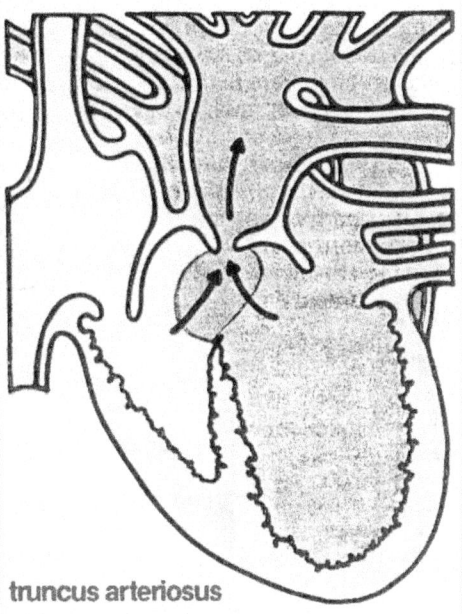

truncus arteriosus

TYPE A BEHAVIOR
See Behavior, Type A and Type B.

TYPE B BEHAVIOR
See Behavior, Type A and Type B.

U

ULTRASOUND *(ul'tra-sownd)*
High frequency sound vibrations, not audible to the human ear. In a sonar-like application, it can be used by cardiologists for diagnosis. **See Echocardiography.**

UNSATURATED FAT *(un-sat'u-rat"ed)*
A fat whose molecules have one or more double bonds, so that it is capable of absorbing more hydrogen. **Mono-unsaturated fats,** such as olive oil, have only one double bond (the rest are single) and seem to have little effect on blood cholesterol. **Polyunsaturated fats,** such as corn oil and safflower oil, have two or more double bonds per molecule and tend to lower blood cholesterol. **See Saturated Fat.**

V

VAGUS NERVES *(va'gus)*
Two of the nerves of the parasympathetic nervous system which extend from the brain, through the neck and thorax into the abdomen. Known as the inhibitory nerves of the heart, they slow the heart rate when stimulated.

VALVE
A flap of tissue which prevents backflow of blood to keep it moving through the heart and circulatory system in the right direction. There are tiny valves along the inside of the veins and four large valves at the entrances and exits of the ventricles in the heart. **See Aortic, Mitral, Pulmonary, and Tricuspid Valves.**

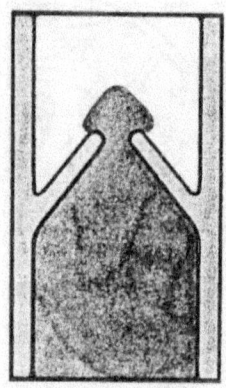 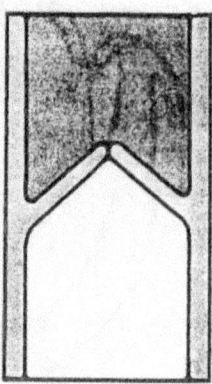

how a one-way valve works

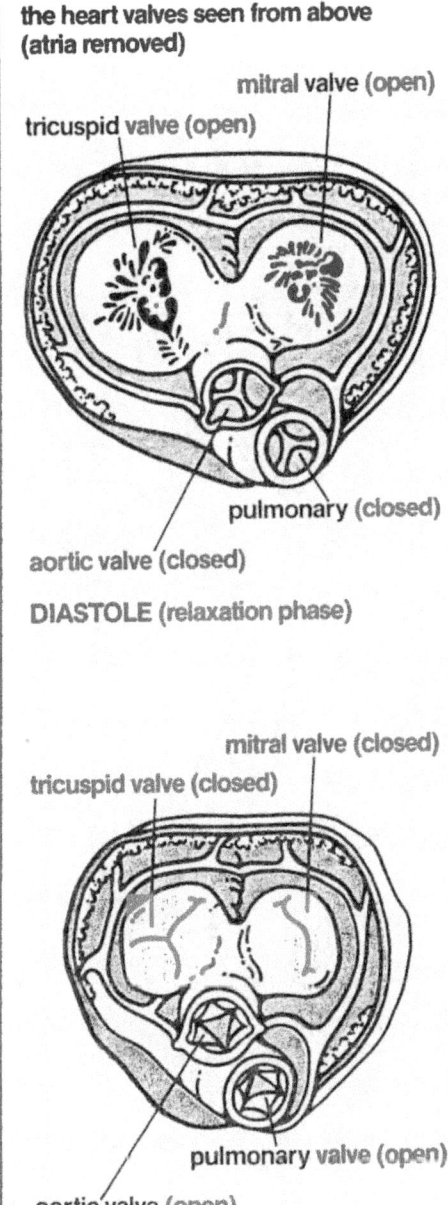

the heart valves seen from above (atria removed)

DIASTOLE (relaxation phase)

SYSTOLE (contraction phase)

right side   left side

VALVULAR INSUFFICIENCY *(val'vu-lar)*
Valves which close improperly and permit a backflow of blood in the wrong direction. **See Incompetent Valve.**

VARICOSE VEINS *(var'i-kos)*
Also called "varicosities" and "varices," they are swollen veins found most frequently on the legs, especially the calves. **See Varix.**

VARIX *(var'iks)*
A varicosity or abnormally swollen vein, artery, or lymph vessel. The plural form is "varices." Varices can occur in such locations as the esophagus, the anus, or the legs (where they are more commonly called "varicose veins"). **See Esophageal Varices, Hemorrhoids, and Varicose Veins.**

VASCULAR *(vas'ku-lar)*
Pertaining to the blood vessels.

VASO- *(vas'o)*
A combining form meaning vessel or duct.

VASOCONSTRICTOR *(vas"o-kon-strik'tor)*
Vasoconstrictor nerves are a part of the involuntary nervous system. When these nerves are stimulated, they cause the muscles of the arterioles to contract, narrowing the arteriole passage, increasing the resistance to bloodflow, and raising the blood pressure.

Vasoconstrictor agents (or vasopressors) are chemical substances which stimulate the muscles of the arterioles to contract. An example is norepinephrine (noradrenalin).

VASODILATOR *(vas"o-di-lat'or)*
Vasodilator nerves are certain nerve fibers of the involuntary nervous system which cause the muscle of the arterioles to relax, thus enlarging the arteriole passage, reducing resistance to the flow of blood, and lowering blood pressure.

Vasodilator agents are chemical compounds which cause a relaxation of the muscles of the arterioles. Examples are nitroglycerin and other nitrites, hydralazine, and many others.

VASOINHIBITOR *(vas"o-in-hib'i-tor)*
An agent which inhibits the action of the vasomotor nerves, that is, an agent which prevents the blood vessels from a normal response (constriction or dilation) to stimuli.

VASOMOTOR *(vas"o-mo'tor)*
Any agent (nerve or substance) that affects the caliber of a vessel, especially of a blood vessel, that is, any agent that is either a vasoconstrictor or a vasodilator.

VASOPRESSOR *(vas"o-pres'or)*
A vasoconstrictor agent. **See Vasoconstrictor and also Pressor.**

VECTORCARDIOGRAPHY *(vek"tor-kar"de-og'rah-fe)*
Determination of the direction and magnitude of the electrical forces of the heart by using electrocardiography in three dimensions.

VEIN *(vain)*
Any one of a series of vessels of the vascular system which carries blood from various parts of the body back to the heart. All veins in the body conduct unoxygenated blood except the pulmonary veins which conduct freshly oxygenated blood from the lungs back to the heart.

VENA CAVA *(ve'nah ka'vah)*
One of the two great veins which conduct unoxygenated blood from the body to the right atrium of the heart. The superior vena cava brings blood from the upper part of the body (head, neck and chest). The inferior vena cava brings blood from the lower part of the body (legs and abdomen). Plural form is **Venae Cavae** *(ve'ni ka'vi)*.

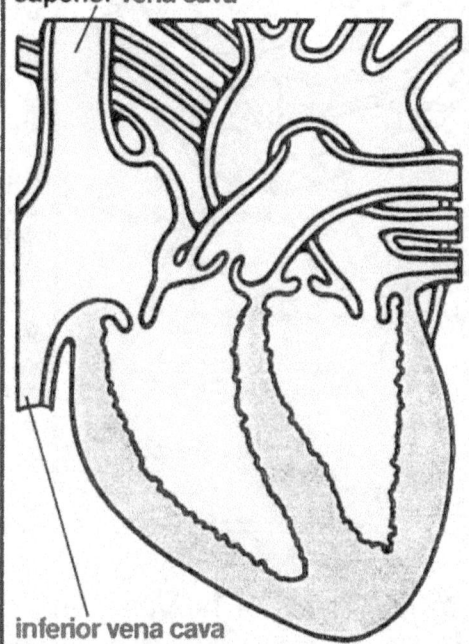

superior vena cava

inferior vena cava

VENOUS BLOOD *(ve'nus)*
Unoxygenated blood. The blood, with hemoglobin in the reduced state, is carried by the veins from all parts of the body back to the heart and then pumped by the right side of the heart through the pulmonary artery to the lungs where it is oxygenated.

VENTRICLE *(ven'tre-kl)*
One of the two main pumping chambers of the heart. The left ventricle pumps oxygenated blood through the arteries to the body. The right ventricle pumps unoxygenated blood through the pulmonary artery to the lungs. Capacity of each ventricle in an adult averages 85 cc. or about 3 ounces.

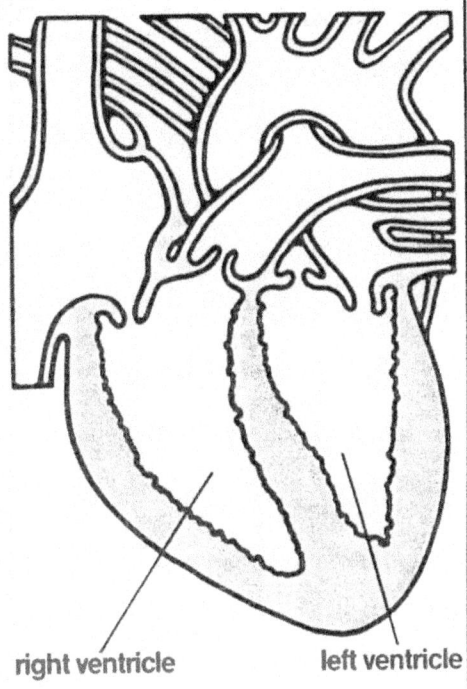

right ventricle   left ventricle

VESALIUS, ANDREAS (1514-1564)
Belgian anatomist who questioned many of the then current theories of the circulatory system as taught by Galen, chiefly the existence of openings in the wall dividing the left from the right side of the heart through which blood was believed to pass.

VISCERAL PERICARDIUM *(vis'er-al per"i-kar'de-um)*
The inner wall of the pericardium, the double-walled sac which surrounds the heart. The visceral pericardium closely adheres to the heart and forms the outermost layer of the heart wall and is also called the epicardium. **For illustration see Pericardium.**

W

WHITE BLOOD CELLS
One of the three kinds of formed elements found in the blood. There are various types of white blood cells. Their best-known function is defense: they destroy foreign bodies, such as bacteria, in areas of infection. Also called leukocytes. **See Red Blood Cells and Platelets.**

WITHERING, WILLIAM (1741-1799)
Eminent English clinician who discovered the use and proper dosage of digitalis in the treatment of heart disease. By analyzing the effective herbal mixture used by an old woman in Shropshire, he identified foxglove leaves as the active ingredient which influenced the function of the heart and kidneys.

WORK CLASSIFICATION UNIT
A community facility involving a team approach to assessing the ability of the cardiac patient to work in terms of the energy requirements of the job.

X

XANTHINE *(zan'theen)*
A class of drugs used among other things to increase the excretion of urine. A diuretic.

XANTHOMA *(zan-tho'mah)*
A new growth of skin occurring as small flat or slightly raised patches or nodules which are yellowish-orange in color. The various types of xanthomas are due to blood lipid disorders (hyperlipoproteinemias).

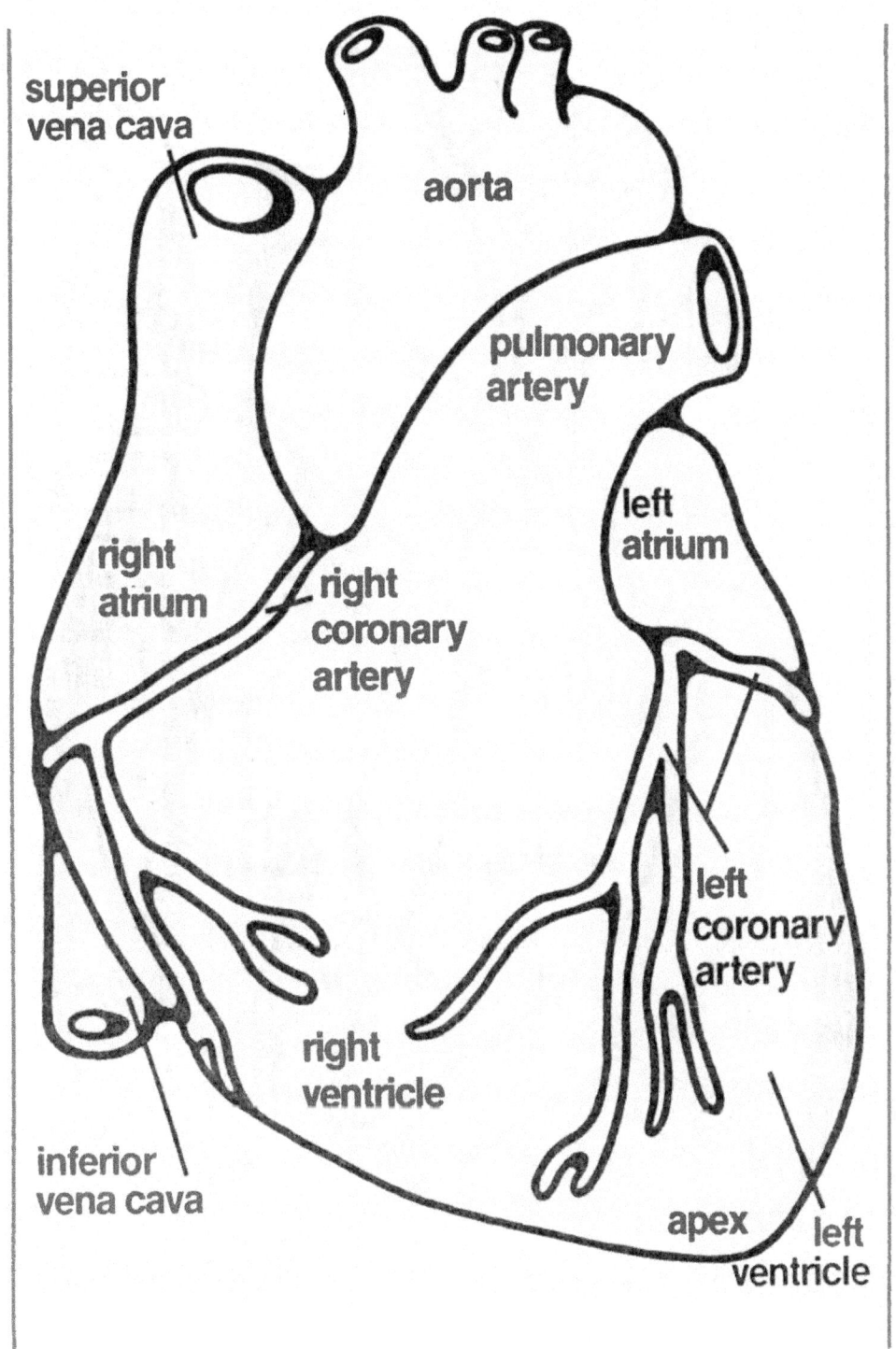

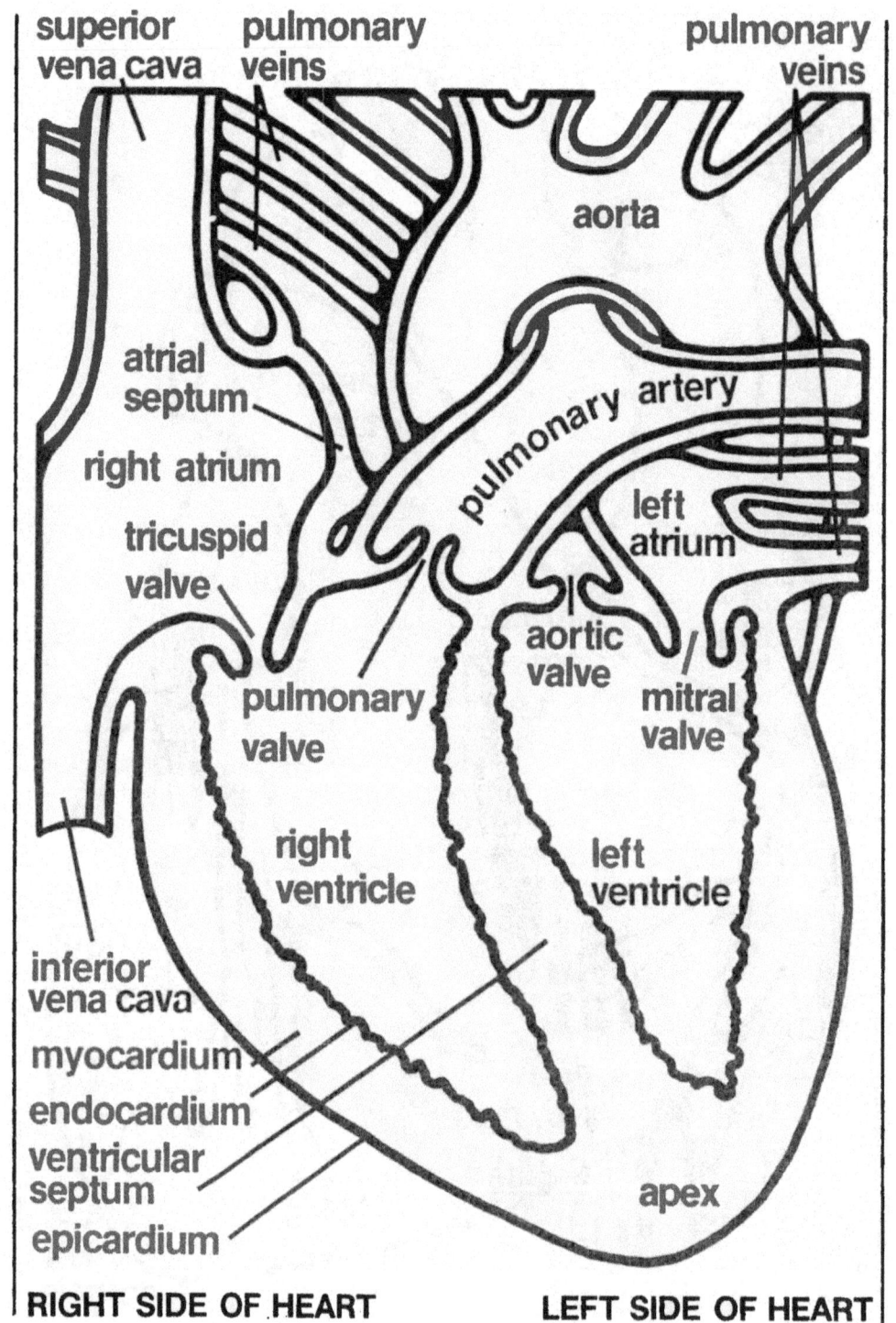

www.ingramcontent.com/pod-product-compliance
Lightning Source LLC
Chambersburg PA
CBHW081808300426
44116CB00014B/2280